SYMPTOMS MATTER!

A WORKBOOK TO RECORD & TRACK YOUR SYMPTOMS TO SHOW YOU WHERE YOU CAN IMPROVE YOUR HEALTH

Compiled by Charlotte Fox

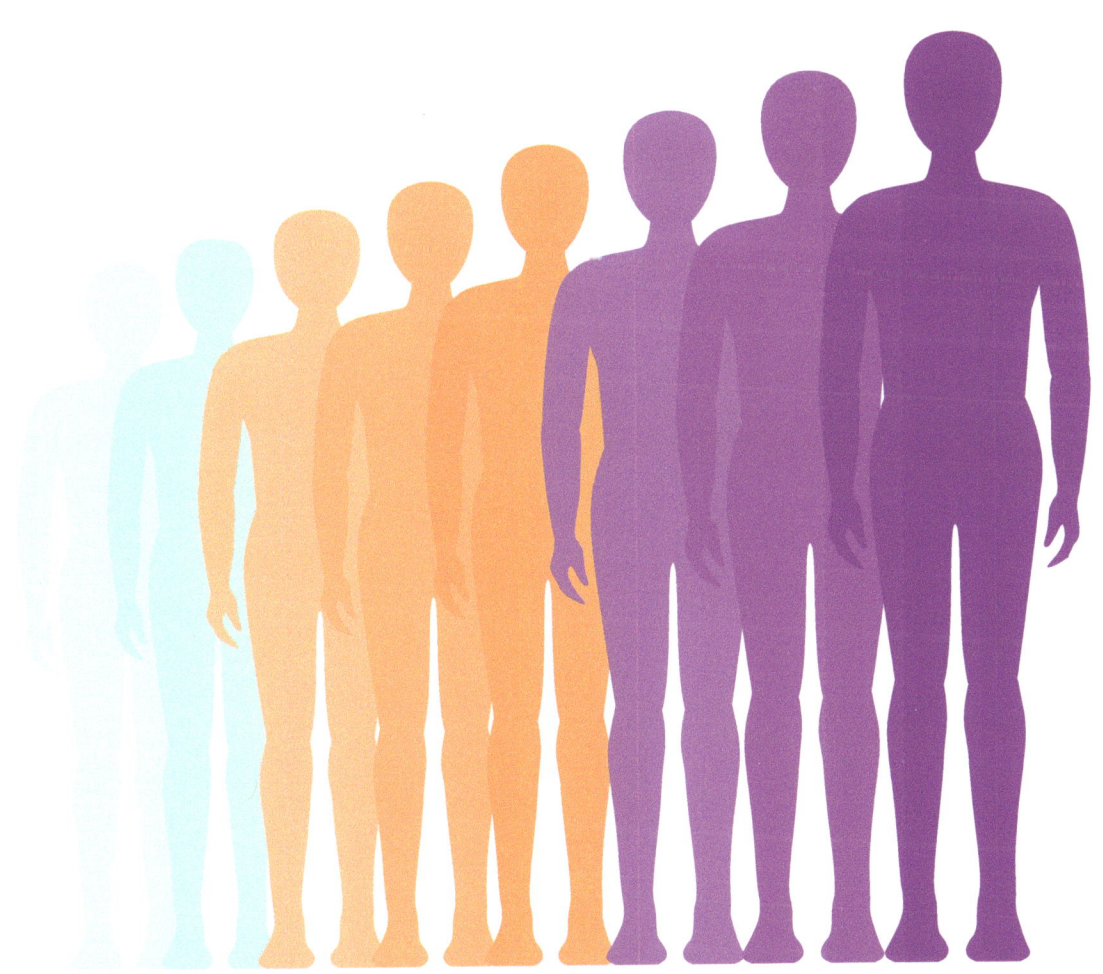

WITH FOREWORD BY DR. CARRIE BURNETT-STRONG

SYMPTOMS MATTER!

A WORKBOOK TO RECORD
AND TRACK YOUR SYMPTOMS
TO SHOW YOU WHERE
YOU CAN IMPROVE YOUR HEALTH

© 2021 Charlotte Fox
ISBN 978-0-9861530-6-8

All rights reserved. No portion of this book may be reproduced for any reason, at any time, in any form, without permission from the author.

Published by Fox Publications LLC
Flagstaff, Arizona

www.therewasone.com
E-mail: FoxPublications1@gmail.com

Nation of Publication: United States

Graphic Design and Editing

Andi Kleinman
Flagstaff, Arizona

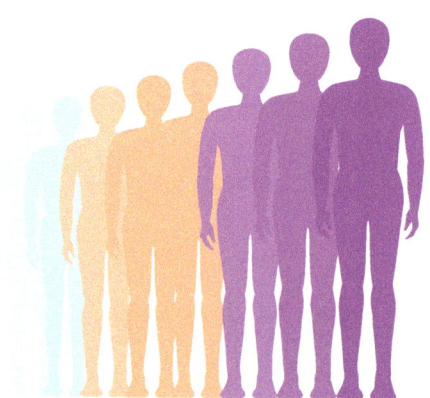

DISCLAIMER: SYMPTOMS MATTER! is a workbook designed for a patient/caregiver to record daily health information to be shared with healthcare professionals. This workbook is not intended to give medical advice and it is not meant to substitute for regular consultations with your healthcare professionals.

FOREWORD

Dear Reader,

This workbook is an excellent source for recording and tracking health symptoms.

So many symptoms are subtle, overlooked, or discounted. The **SYMPTOMS MATTER!** workbook will bring them to mind in a logical way that anyone can record, track, and take to their doctor(s) and/or heathcare practitioner(s). I look forward to my patients using this workbook.

Thank you Charlotte, for being so very good at this!

Sincerely,

Dr. Carrie Burnett-Strong

Dr. Carrie Burnett-Strong
Cedar Chiropractic
Flagstaff, Arizona

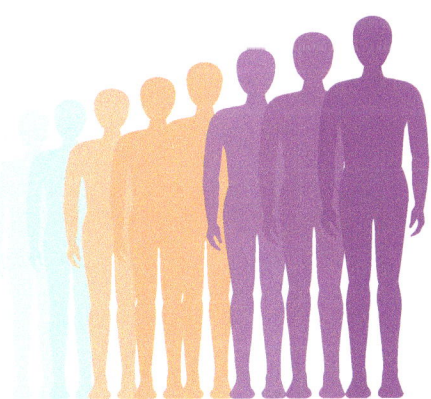

THIS WORKBOOK BELONGS TO

_____

My Contact Info

_____

_____

ABOUT THE SYMPTOMS MATTER! WORKBOOK

The SYMPTOMS MATTER! workbook is self-explanatory. Within these pages, you will find two months' worth of sheets to record your daily health-related symptoms—from blood pressure to how you slept the night before, and everything in between.

At the end of each orange and purple section, there are lined summary pages where you can record additional positive or negative reactions to food, perfumes, soaps, household cleaning products, etc., and anything else that jumps out at you worth noting.

To get the best benefit and overview of your health, be honest and thorough when completing the entries.

Keep the SYMPTOMS MATTER! workbook (and a supply of pens and pencils) in a handy place where it will be easy to grab and write in it. For more convenience, add a ribbon or a bookmark to keep your place. An office supply store can 3-hole-punch the workbook or add a spiral binding for you if you wish.

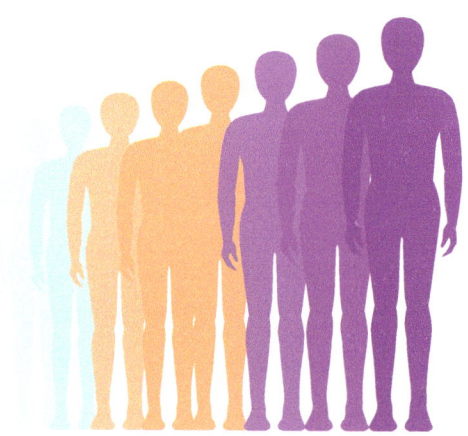

A LETTER FROM THE AUTHOR

Dear Friends:

For decades I dealt with various health challenges…conditions that were debilitating to say the least! My health practitioners always asked me about my symptoms, environment, food intake, supplements, bathroom experiences, sleep habits, if I had dreams, etc. Because I couldn't remember, (yet another symptom), I was forced to start writing everything down. I was intimidated at first, but soon discovered that a written record is a very useful tool.

You may wonder if you have the discipline to fill in the blanks every day. Trust me—you do! When you see how worthwhile it is—and that it's only for a short period of time—you'll realize it's easier than you thought.

The knowledge you gain from completing the workbook is eye-opening. You'll be able to see at a glance what affects you and say, "Aha! that's why that happened;" or, "That's what made me feel that way;" or, "I best not do THAT again." Some symptoms are immediate… some take a day or two or longer to manifest. Whatever the case, *your body will hold you accountable to whatever you do; it's to your benefit to pay attention to it!*

By keeping a record of what you do, your environment, *and what goes in and out of your body,* you will discover a new commitment to your health. Uncovering which activities, environmental factors, foods, and drinks have positive and negative effects on your health may be a huge wake-up call for you.

A filled-in **SYMPTOMS MATTER!** workbook will make your healthcare practitioners' job much easier. Although they may adhere to different disciplines and approaches, it will present a more comprehensive picture of your health. And, by pinpointing your underlying health factors, they will be more likely to diagnose your condition(s) more accurately, and treat you as a whole person—not just your symptoms.

Positive change takes time. The **SYMPTOMS MATTER!** workbook gives you two months in which to help you develop life-improving habits.

I wish you happiness and new-found good health.

Warm Regards,

Charlotte

Charlotte Fox
Flagstaff, Arizona

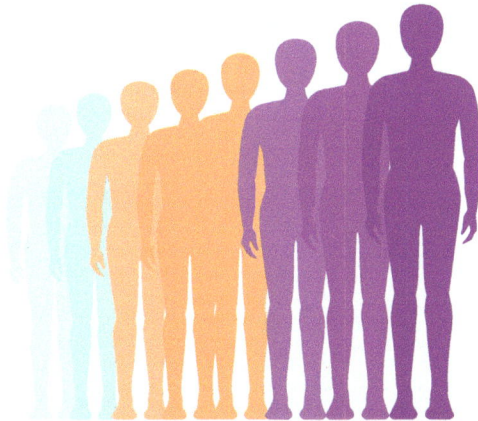

HEALTHCARE PROFESSIONALS / DENTISTS / THERAPISTS / ETC.

Name: _____ Phone: _____

Specialty: _____ Patient Portal: _____

Address: _____ Office Contact: _____

Name: _____ Phone: _____

Specialty: _____ Patient Portal: _____

Address: _____ Office Contact: _____

Name: _____ Phone: _____

Specialty: _____ Patient Portal: _____

Address: _____ Office Contact: _____

Name: _____ Phone: _____

Specialty: _____ Patient Portal: _____

Address: _____ Office Contact: _____

Name: _____ Phone: _____

Specialty: _____ Patient Portal: _____

Address: _____ Office Contact: _____

WHO TO NOTIFY IN CASE OF EMERGENCY / PHONE NUMBER

_____

_____

WHO TO CALL FOR A RIDE / PHONE NUMBER

_____

_____

HEALTHCARE PROFESSIONALS / DENTISTS / THERAPISTS / ETC.

Name: _____ Phone: _____

Specialty: _____ Patient Portal: _____

Address: _____ Office Contact: _____

Name: _____ Phone: _____

Specialty: _____ Patient Portal: _____

Address: _____ Office Contact: _____

Name: _____ Phone: _____

Specialty: _____ Patient Portal: _____

Address: _____ Office Contact: _____

Name: _____ Phone: _____

Specialty: _____ Patient Portal: _____

Address: _____ Office Contact: _____

Name: _____ Phone: _____

Specialty: _____ Patient Portal: _____

Address: _____ Office Contact: _____

HOSPICE INFORMATION

Name of Hospice: _____ Phone: _____

Contact: _____ Phone: _____

Caregiver: _____ Phone: _____

Days & Times for Hospice Visits:

☐ Sun ☐ Mon ☐ Tue ☐ Wed ☐ Thur ☐ Fri ☐ Sat

_____

SYMPTOMS MATTER!

Here are a few symptoms worth noting on your daily pages. Jot down these (and/or others) that apply to you.

Acne	Eczema	Neck Can't Support Head
Allergies	Eye Problems	Paralysis
Bad Breath	Fatigue	Perspiring
Belly Bloat/Gas	Fever	Runny Nose
Body Odor	Fuzzy Focus	Sad/Depressed
Body/Muscle Pain	Gassy	Shaky
Brain Fog	Gassy with Pain	Shortness of Breath
Breathing Difficulties	Headaches	Sinus Pain
Bruise Easily	Heart Problems	Skin Problems
Chemical Sensitivities	Heartburn	Sleep Problems
Cold Hands, Feet, Nose	Heavy Legs and Arms	Sore Throat
Constipation	Itchy	Things Smell Like Vinegar
Cramps	Joint Pain	Thirsty
Cravings	Low/High Blood Pressure	Tongue Issues
Dehydrated	Memory Problems	Tooth & Gum Issues
Dizziness	Muscle Weakness	Vision Problems
Drop Things Often	Nausea	Vomiting, When Sick (or not)

CONDITION / DIAGNOSES CURRENTLY ADDRESSING

_____
_____
_____
_____
_____
_____
_____

DRUG, FOOD, & OTHER ALLERGIES

DAILY PRESCRIPTIONS & SUPPLEMENTS (WITH DOSAGES)

IMMUNIZATIONS & VACCINATIONS

ADDITIONAL TREATMENTS (INJECTIONS, IVS, ETC.)

BLOOD PRESSURE

Date Range: _____ to _____ .

Date	Reading	Hour/Minute

Date	Reading	Hour/Minute

OXIMETER

Date Range: _____ to _____ .

Date	Oxygen	Pulse	Hour/Minute	Date	Oxygen	Pulse	Hour/Minute

| TEMP | **TODAY'S SLEEP** |

Last night, I went to bed at _____   Today, I woke up at _____

I fell asleep at _____ ☐ Dreams?   I felt   ☐ Rested & ready for the day

I slept ☐ Well   ☐ Restless   ☐ Insomnia   ☐ Stiff ☐ Tired ☐ Sick ☐ Sore ☐ Pain

I got up _____ times to _____   Describe _____

TODAY'S PRESCRIPTIONS AND/OR SUPPLEMENTS*

Time	Prescription/Supplement	Time	Prescription/Supplement

*NOTE: WHAT YOU APPLY TO YOUR SKIN MATTERS TOO!

TODAY'S EXERCISE

Type	Time	Distance, Pounds, Repetitions, etc.
Walking		
Running		
Cycling		
Stretching		

TODAY'S ACCOMPLISHMENTS (NO MATTER HOW INSIGNIFICANT THEY MAY SEEM)

_____

_____

_____

WEIGHT	TODAY'S RECORD	DATE

Weather: ☐ Sun ☐ Clouds ☐ Rain ☐ Wind ☐ Snow   Barometer:_____   Temp:____/____

I have felt: ☐ Cold   ☐ Hot   ☐ Comfortable   ☐ Mixed-bag   ☐ _____

TODAY'S FOOD & DRINK

Time	Food	How I Felt After Eating

Cravings: ☐ Sweet   ☐ Salty   ☐ Spicy   ☐ Bitter   ☐ _____

Water Consumed: ozs.   (YOUR WEIGHT DIVIDED BY 2, EQUALS [GOAL] OUNCES TO DRINK DAILY.*)

Other Liquids Consumed & How I Felt

*HIGH ELEVATION & CHRONIC-PAIN PATIENTS, CALCULATE 1 QUART WATER PER 50 POUNDS OF WEIGHT.

BATHROOM EXPERIENCES

Bowels ☐ Constipation ☐ Diarrhea	☐ Formed ☐ Pain _____ Times	☐ Loose ☐ Pain _____ Times	☐ Cowpie ☐ Pain _____ Times	☐ Soup ☐ Pain _____ Times	☐ Odor? ☐ Painful Gas _____ Times
Urine ☐ Too Often ☐ Infrequent	☐ Clear ☐ Pain _____ Times	☐ Cloudy ☐ Pain _____ Times	☐ Light Yellow ☐ Pain _____ Times	☐ Dark Yellow ☐ Pain _____ Times	☐ Odor? ☐ Pain _____ Times

BASAL* TEMPERATURE / BLOOD-SUGAR NUMBERS / NOTES / ETC.

*The temperature that registers on an oral thermometer when it is placed under the armpit first thing in the morning before any activity.

NOTE: Your regular body temperature (TEMP) is written in the oval on the top of the left-hand side.

TEMP

TODAY'S SLEEP

Last night, I went to bed at _____ Today, I woke up at _____

I fell asleep at _____ ☐ Dreams? I felt ☐ Rested & ready for the day

I slept ☐ Well ☐ Restless ☐ Insomnia ☐ Stiff ☐ Tired ☐ Sick ☐ Sore ☐ Pain

I got up _____ times to _____ Describe _____

TODAY'S PRESCRIPTIONS AND/OR SUPPLEMENTS*

Time	Prescription/Supplement	Time	Prescription/Supplement

*NOTE: WHAT YOU APPLY TO YOUR SKIN MATTERS TOO!

TODAY'S EXERCISE

Type	Time	Distance, Pounds, Repetitions, etc.
Walking		
Running		
Cycling		
Stretching		

TODAY'S ACCOMPLISHMENTS (NO MATTER HOW INSIGNIFICANT THEY MAY SEEM)

_____

_____

_____

| WEIGHT | TODAY'S RECORD | DATE |

Weather: ☐ Sun ☐ Clouds ☐ Rain ☐ Wind ☐ Snow   Barometer:_____   Temp:____ / ____

I have felt: ☐ Cold   ☐ Hot   ☐ Comfortable   ☐ Mixed-bag   ☐ _____

TODAY'S FOOD & DRINK

Time	Food	How I Felt After Eating

Cravings: ☐ Sweet   ☐ Salty   ☐ Spicy   ☐ Bitter   ☐ _____

Water Consumed: _____ ozs.   (YOUR WEIGHT DIVIDED BY 2, EQUALS [GOAL] OUNCES TO DRINK DAILY.*)

Other Liquids Consumed & How I Felt

*HIGH ELEVATION & CHRONIC-PAIN PATIENTS, CALCULATE 1 QUART WATER PER 50 POUNDS OF WEIGHT.

BATHROOM EXPERIENCES

Bowels ☐ Constipation ☐ Diarrhea	☐ Formed ☐ Pain _____ Times	☐ Loose ☐ Pain _____ Times	☐ Cowpie ☐ Pain _____ Times	☐ Soup ☐ Pain _____ Times	☐ Odor? ☐ Painful Gas _____ Times
Urine ☐ Too Often ☐ Infrequent	☐ Clear ☐ Pain _____ Times	☐ Cloudy ☐ Pain _____ Times	☐ Light Yellow ☐ Pain _____ Times	☐ Dark Yellow ☐ Pain _____ Times	☐ Odor? ☐ Pain _____ Times

BASAL* TEMPERATURE / BLOOD-SUGAR NUMBERS / NOTES / ETC.

*The temperature that registers on an oral thermometer when it is placed under the armpit first thing in the morning before any activity.

NOTE: Your regular body temperature (TEMP) is written in the oval on the top of the left-hand side.

| TEMP | **TODAY'S SLEEP** |

Last night, I went to bed at _____   Today, I woke up at _____

I fell asleep at _____ ☐ Dreams?   I felt ☐ Rested & ready for the day

I slept ☐ Well ☐ Restless ☐ Insomnia   ☐ Stiff ☐ Tired ☐ Sick ☐ Sore ☐ Pain

I got up _____ times to _____   Describe _____

TODAY'S PRESCRIPTIONS AND/OR SUPPLEMENTS*

Time	Prescription/Supplement	Time	Prescription/Supplement

*NOTE: WHAT YOU APPLY TO YOUR SKIN MATTERS TOO!

TODAY'S EXERCISE

Type	Time	Distance, Pounds, Repetitions, etc.
Walking		
Running		
Cycling		
Stretching		

TODAY'S ACCOMPLISHMENTS (NO MATTER HOW INSIGNIFICANT THEY MAY SEEM)

_____

_____

_____

| WEIGHT | TODAY'S RECORD | DATE |

Weather: ☐ Sun ☐ Clouds ☐ Rain ☐ Wind ☐ Snow   Barometer:_____   Temp:____ H / L

I have felt: ☐ Cold   ☐ Hot   ☐ Comfortable   ☐ Mixed-bag   ☐ _____

TODAY'S FOOD & DRINK

Time	Food	How I Felt After Eating

Cravings: ☐ Sweet   ☐ Salty   ☐ Spicy   ☐ Bitter   ☐ _____

Water Consumed: _____ OZS. (YOUR WEIGHT DIVIDED BY 2, EQUALS [GOAL] OUNCES TO DRINK DAILY.*)

Other Liquids Consumed & How I Felt

*HIGH ELEVATION & CHRONIC-PAIN PATIENTS, CALCULATE 1 QUART WATER PER 50 POUNDS OF WEIGHT.

BATHROOM EXPERIENCES

Bowels ☐ Constipation ☐ Diarrhea	☐ Formed ☐ Pain ____ Times	☐ Loose ☐ Pain ____ Times	☐ Cowpie ☐ Pain ____ Times	☐ Soup ☐ Pain ____ Times	☐ Odor? ☐ Painful Gas ____ Times
Urine ☐ Too Often ☐ Infrequent	☐ Clear ☐ Pain ____ Times	☐ Cloudy ☐ Pain ____ Times	☐ Light Yellow ☐ Pain ____ Times	☐ Dark Yellow ☐ Pain ____ Times	☐ Odor? ☐ Pain ____ Times

BASAL* TEMPERATURE / BLOOD-SUGAR NUMBERS / NOTES / ETC.

*The temperature that registers on an oral thermometer when it is placed under the armpit first thing in the morning before any activity.

NOTE: Your regular body temperature (TEMP) is written in the oval on the top of the left-hand side.

(TEMP)

TODAY'S SLEEP

Last night, I went to bed at _____

I fell asleep at _____ ☐ Dreams?

I slept ☐ Well ☐ Restless ☐ Insomnia

I got up _____ times to _____

Today, I woke up at _____

I felt ☐ Rested & ready for the day

☐ Stiff ☐ Tired ☐ Sick ☐ Sore ☐ Pain

Describe _____

TODAY'S PRESCRIPTIONS AND/OR SUPPLEMENTS*

Time	Prescription/Supplement	Time	Prescription/Supplement

*NOTE: WHAT YOU APPLY TO YOUR SKIN MATTERS TOO!

TODAY'S EXERCISE

Type	Time	Distance, Pounds, Repetitions, etc.
Walking		
Running		
Cycling		
Stretching		

TODAY'S ACCOMPLISHMENTS (NO MATTER HOW INSIGNIFICANT THEY MAY SEEM)

_____

_____

_____

WEIGHT	TODAY'S RECORD	DATE

Weather: ☐ Sun ☐ Clouds ☐ Rain ☐ Wind ☐ Snow   Barometer:_____   Temp:____/____

I have felt: ☐ Cold   ☐ Hot   ☐ Comfortable   ☐ Mixed-bag   ☐ _____

TODAY'S FOOD & DRINK

Time	Food	How I Felt After Eating

Cravings: ☐ Sweet   ☐ Salty   ☐ Spicy   ☐ Bitter   ☐ _____

Water Consumed: ozs.   (YOUR WEIGHT DIVIDED BY 2, EQUALS [GOAL] OUNCES TO DRINK DAILY.*)

Other Liquids Consumed & How I Felt

*HIGH ELEVATION & CHRONIC-PAIN PATIENTS, CALCULATE 1 QUART WATER PER 50 POUNDS OF WEIGHT.

BATHROOM EXPERIENCES

Bowels ☐ Constipation ☐ Diarrhea	☐ Formed ☐ Pain _____ Times	☐ Loose ☐ Pain _____ Times	☐ Cowpie ☐ Pain _____ Times	☐ Soup ☐ Pain _____ Times	☐ Odor? ☐ Painful Gas _____ Times
Urine ☐ Too Often ☐ Infrequent	☐ Clear ☐ Pain _____ Times	☐ Cloudy ☐ Pain _____ Times	☐ Light Yellow ☐ Pain _____ Times	☐ Dark Yellow ☐ Pain _____ Times	☐ Odor? ☐ Pain _____ Times

BASAL* TEMPERATURE / BLOOD-SUGAR NUMBERS / NOTES / ETC.

*The temperature that registers on an oral thermometer when it is placed under the armpit first thing in the morning before any activity.

NOTE: Your regular body temperature (TEMP) is written in the oval on the top of the left-hand side.

TEMP

TODAY'S SLEEP

Last night, I went to bed at _____ Today, I woke up at _____

I fell asleep at _____ ☐ Dreams? I felt ☐ Rested & ready for the day

I slept ☐ Well ☐ Restless ☐ Insomnia ☐ Stiff ☐ Tired ☐ Sick ☐ Sore ☐ Pain

I got up _____ times to _____ Describe _____

TODAY'S PRESCRIPTIONS AND/OR SUPPLEMENTS*

Time	Prescription/Supplement	Time	Prescription/Supplement

*NOTE: WHAT YOU APPLY TO YOUR SKIN MATTERS TOO!

TODAY'S EXERCISE

Type	Time	Distance, Pounds, Repetitions, etc.
Walking		
Running		
Cycling		
Stretching		

TODAY'S ACCOMPLISHMENTS (NO MATTER HOW INSIGNIFICANT THEY MAY SEEM)

_____

_____

_____

WEIGHT	TODAY'S RECORD	DATE

Weather: ☐ Sun ☐ Clouds ☐ Rain ☐ Wind ☐ Snow   Barometer:_____   Temp:___H_/_L_

I have felt: ☐ Cold   ☐ Hot   ☐ Comfortable   ☐ Mixed-bag   ☐_____

TODAY'S FOOD & DRINK

Time	Food	How I Felt After Eating

Cravings: ☐ Sweet   ☐ Salty   ☐ Spicy   ☐ Bitter   ☐_____

Water Consumed: OZS. (YOUR WEIGHT DIVIDED BY 2, EQUALS [GOAL] OUNCES TO DRINK DAILY.*)

Other Liquids Consumed & How I Felt

^HIGH ELEVATION & CHRONIC-PAIN PATIENTS, CALCULATE 1 QUART WATER PER 50 POUNDS OF WEIGHT.

BATHROOM EXPERIENCES

Bowels ☐ Constipation ☐ Diarrhea	☐ Formed ☐ Pain _____ Times	☐ Loose ☐ Pain _____ Times	☐ Cowpie ☐ Pain _____ Times	☐ Soup ☐ Pain _____ Times	☐ Odor? ☐ Painful Gas _____ Times
Urine ☐ Too Often ☐ Infrequent	☐ Clear ☐ Pain _____ Times	☐ Cloudy ☐ Pain _____ Times	☐ Light Yellow ☐ Pain _____ Times	☐ Dark Yellow ☐ Pain _____ Times	☐ Odor? ☐ Pain _____ Times

BASAL* TEMPERATURE / BLOOD-SUGAR NUMBERS / NOTES / ETC.

*The temperature that registers on an oral thermometer when it is placed under the armpit first thing in the morning before any activity.

NOTE: Your regular body temperature (TEMP) is written in the oval on the top of the left-hand side.

(TEMP)

TODAY'S SLEEP

Last night, I went to bed at _____

I fell asleep at _____ ☐ Dreams?

I slept ☐ Well   ☐ Restless   ☐ Insomnia

I got up _____ times to _____

Today, I woke up at _____

I felt ☐ Rested & ready for the day

☐ Stiff   ☐ Tired   ☐ Sick   ☐ Sore   ☐ Pain

Describe _____

TODAY'S PRESCRIPTIONS AND/OR SUPPLEMENTS*

Time	Prescription/Supplement	Time	Prescription/Supplement

*NOTE: WHAT YOU APPLY TO YOUR SKIN MATTERS TOO!

TODAY'S EXERCISE

Type	Time	Distance, Pounds, Repetitions, etc.
Walking		
Running		
Cycling		
Stretching		

TODAY'S ACCOMPLISHMENTS (NO MATTER HOW INSIGNIFICANT THEY MAY SEEM)

_____

_____

_____

WEIGHT	TODAY'S RECORD	DATE

Weather: ☐ Sun ☐ Clouds ☐ Rain ☐ Wind ☐ Snow   Barometer:_____   Temp:_____

I have felt: ☐ Cold ☐ Hot ☐ Comfortable ☐ Mixed-bag ☐ _____

TODAY'S FOOD & DRINK

Time	Food	How I Felt After Eating

Cravings: ☐ Sweet ☐ Salty ☐ Spicy ☐ Bitter ☐ _____

Water Consumed: OZS. (YOUR WEIGHT DIVIDED BY 2, EQUALS [GOAL] OUNCES TO DRINK DAILY.*)

Other Liquids Consumed & How I Felt

*HIGH ELEVATION & CHRONIC-PAIN PATIENTS, CALCULATE 1 QUART WATER PER 50 POUNDS OF WEIGHT.

BATHROOM EXPERIENCES

Bowels ☐ Constipation ☐ Diarrhea	☐ Formed ☐ Pain _____ Times	☐ Loose ☐ Pain _____ Times	☐ Cowpie ☐ Pain _____ Times	☐ Soup ☐ Pain _____ Times	☐ Odor? ☐ Painful Gas _____ Times
Urine ☐ Too Often ☐ Infrequent	☐ Clear ☐ Pain _____ Times	☐ Cloudy ☐ Pain _____ Times	☐ Light Yellow ☐ Pain _____ Times	☐ Dark Yellow ☐ Pain _____ Times	☐ Odor? ☐ Pain _____ Times

BASAL* TEMPERATURE / BLOOD-SUGAR NUMBERS / NOTES / ETC.

*The temperature that registers on an oral thermometer when it is placed under the armpit first thing in the morning before any activity.

NOTE: Your regular body temperature (TEMP) is written in the oval on the top of the left-hand side.

TEMP		

TODAY'S SLEEP

Last night, I went to bed at _____ Today, I woke up at _____

I fell asleep at _____ ☐ Dreams? I felt ☐ Rested & ready for the day

I slept ☐ Well ☐ Restless ☐ Insomnia ☐ Stiff ☐ Tired ☐ Sick ☐ Sore ☐ Pain

I got up _____ times to _____ Describe _____

TODAY'S PRESCRIPTIONS AND/OR SUPPLEMENTS*

Time	Prescription/Supplement	Time	Prescription/Supplement

*NOTE: WHAT YOU APPLY TO YOUR SKIN MATTERS TOO!

TODAY'S EXERCISE

Type	Time	Distance, Pounds, Repetitions, etc.
Walking		
Running		
Cycling		
Stretching		

TODAY'S ACCOMPLISHMENTS (NO MATTER HOW INSIGNIFICANT THEY MAY SEEM)

_____

_____

_____

| WEIGHT | TODAY'S RECORD | DATE |

Weather: ☐ Sun ☐ Clouds ☐ Rain ☐ Wind ☐ Snow   Barometer:_____   Temp:___H_/_L_

I have felt: ☐ Cold   ☐ Hot   ☐ Comfortable   ☐ Mixed-bag   ☐ _____

TODAY'S FOOD & DRINK

Time	Food	How I Felt After Eating

Cravings: ☐ Sweet   ☐ Salty   ☐ Spicy   ☐ Bitter   ☐ _____

Water Consumed: OZS.   (YOUR WEIGHT DIVIDED BY 2, EQUALS [GOAL] OUNCES TO DRINK DAILY.*)

Other Liquids Consumed & How I Felt

*HIGH ELEVATION & CHRONIC-PAIN PATIENTS, CALCULATE 1 QUART WATER PER 50 POUNDS OF WEIGHT.

BATHROOM EXPERIENCES

Bowels ☐ Constipation ☐ Diarrhea	☐ Formed ☐ Pain _____ Times	☐ Loose ☐ Pain _____ Times	☐ Cowpie ☐ Pain _____ Times	☐ Soup ☐ Pain _____ Times	☐ Odor? ☐ Painful Gas _____ Times
Urine ☐ Too Often ☐ Infrequent	☐ Clear ☐ Pain _____ Times	☐ Cloudy ☐ Pain _____ Times	☐ Light Yellow ☐ Pain _____ Times	☐ Dark Yellow ☐ Pain _____ Times	☐ Odor? ☐ Pain _____ Times

BASAL* TEMPERATURE / BLOOD-SUGAR NUMBERS / NOTES / ETC.

*The temperature that registers on an oral thermometer when it is placed under the armpit first thing in the morning before any activity.

NOTE: Your regular body temperature (TEMP) is written in the oval on the top of the left-hand side.

TEMP	TODAY'S SLEEP	
Last night, I went to bed at _____		Today, I woke up at _____
I fell asleep at _____ ☐ Dreams?		I felt ☐ Rested & ready for the day
I slept ☐ Well ☐ Restless ☐ Insomnia		☐ Stiff ☐ Tired ☐ Sick ☐ Sore ☐ Pain
I got up _____ times to _____		Describe _____

TODAY'S PRESCRIPTIONS AND/OR SUPPLEMENTS*

Time	Prescription/Supplement	Time	Prescription/Supplement

*NOTE: WHAT YOU APPLY TO YOUR SKIN MATTERS TOO!

TODAY'S EXERCISE

Type	Time	Distance, Pounds, Repetitions, etc.
Walking		
Running		
Cycling		
Stretching		

TODAY'S ACCOMPLISHMENTS (NO MATTER HOW INSIGNIFICANT THEY MAY SEEM)

_____

_____

_____

TODAY'S RECORD

WEIGHT **DATE**

Weather: ☐ Sun ☐ Clouds ☐ Rain ☐ Wind ☐ Snow   Barometer:_____   Temp:____ / ____

I have felt: ☐ Cold   ☐ Hot   ☐ Comfortable   ☐ Mixed-bag   ☐ _____

TODAY'S FOOD & DRINK

Time	Food	How I Felt After Eating

Cravings: ☐ Sweet   ☐ Salty   ☐ Spicy   ☐ Bitter   ☐ _____

Water Consumed: ____ ozs. (YOUR WEIGHT DIVIDED BY 2, EQUALS [GOAL] OUNCES TO DRINK DAILY.*)

Other Liquids Consumed & How I Felt

*HIGH ELEVATION & CHRONIC-PAIN PATIENTS, CALCULATE 1 QUART WATER PER 50 POUNDS OF WEIGHT.

BATHROOM EXPERIENCES

Bowels ☐ Constipation ☐ Diarrhea	☐ Formed ☐ Pain ____ Times	☐ Loose ☐ Pain ____ Times	☐ Cowpie ☐ Pain ____ Times	☐ Soup ☐ Pain ____ Times	☐ Odor? ☐ Painful Gas ____ Times
Urine ☐ Too Often ☐ Infrequent	☐ Clear ☐ Pain ____ Times	☐ Cloudy ☐ Pain ____ Times	☐ Light Yellow ☐ Pain ____ Times	☐ Dark Yellow ☐ Pain ____ Times	☐ Odor? ☐ Pain ____ Times

BASAL* TEMPERATURE / BLOOD-SUGAR NUMBERS / NOTES / ETC.

*The temperature that registers on an oral thermometer when it is placed under the armpit first thing in the morning before any activity.

NOTE: Your regular body temperature (TEMP) is written in the oval on the top of the left-hand side.

TEMP	**TODAY'S SLEEP**

Last night, I went to bed at _____   Today, I woke up at _____

I fell asleep at _____ ☐ Dreams?   I felt ☐ Rested & ready for the day

I slept ☐ Well   ☐ Restless   ☐ Insomnia   ☐ Stiff ☐ Tired ☐ Sick ☐ Sore ☐ Pain

I got up _____ times to _____   Describe _____

TODAY'S PRESCRIPTIONS AND/OR SUPPLEMENTS*

Time	Prescription/Supplement	Time	Prescription/Supplement

*NOTE: WHAT YOU APPLY TO YOUR SKIN MATTERS TOO!

TODAY'S EXERCISE

Type	Time	Distance, Pounds, Repetitions, etc.
Walking		
Running		
Cycling		
Stretching		

TODAY'S ACCOMPLISHMENTS (NO MATTER HOW INSIGNIFICANT THEY MAY SEEM)

_____

_____

_____

| WEIGHT | TODAY'S RECORD | DATE |

Weather: ☐ Sun ☐ Clouds ☐ Rain ☐ Wind ☐ Snow   Barometer:_____   Temp:____ / ____

I have felt: ☐ Cold   ☐ Hot   ☐ Comfortable   ☐ Mixed-bag   ☐ _____

TODAY'S FOOD & DRINK

Time	Food	How I Felt After Eating

Cravings: ☐ Sweet   ☐ Salty   ☐ Spicy   ☐ Bitter   ☐ _____

Water Consumed: ozs. (YOUR WEIGHT DIVIDED BY 2, EQUALS [GOAL] OUNCES TO DRINK DAILY.*)

Other Liquids Consumed & How I Felt

*HIGH ELEVATION & CHRONIC-PAIN PATIENTS, CALCULATE 1 QUART WATER PER 50 POUNDS OF WEIGHT.

BATHROOM EXPERIENCES

Bowels ☐ Constipation ☐ Diarrhea	☐ Formed ☐ Pain _____ Times	☐ Loose ☐ Pain _____ Times	☐ Cowpie ☐ Pain _____ Times	☐ Soup ☐ Pain _____ Times	☐ Odor? ☐ Painful Gas _____ Times
Urine ☐ Too Often ☐ Infrequent	☐ Clear ☐ Pain _____ Times	☐ Cloudy ☐ Pain _____ Times	☐ Light Yellow ☐ Pain _____ Times	☐ Dark Yellow ☐ Pain _____ Times	☐ Odor? ☐ Pain _____ Times

BASAL* TEMPERATURE / BLOOD-SUGAR NUMBERS / NOTES / ETC.

*The temperature that registers on an oral thermometer when it is placed under the armpit first thing in the morning before any activity.

NOTE: Your regular body temperature (TEMP) is written in the oval on the top of the left-hand side.

TODAY'S SLEEP

(TEMP)

Last night, I went to bed at _____

I fell asleep at _____ ☐ Dreams?

I slept ☐ Well ☐ Restless ☐ Insomnia

I got up _____ times to _____

Today, I woke up at _____

I felt ☐ Rested & ready for the day

☐ Stiff ☐ Tired ☐ Sick ☐ Sore ☐ Pain

Describe _____

TODAY'S PRESCRIPTIONS AND/OR SUPPLEMENTS*

Time	Prescription/Supplement	Time	Prescription/Supplement

*NOTE: WHAT YOU APPLY TO YOUR SKIN MATTERS TOO!

TODAY'S EXERCISE

Type	Time	Distance, Pounds, Repetitions, etc.
Walking		
Running		
Cycling		
Stretching		

TODAY'S ACCOMPLISHMENTS (NO MATTER HOW INSIGNIFICANT THEY MAY SEEM)

_____

_____

_____

TODAY'S RECORD

WEIGHT 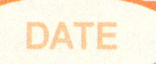 **DATE**

Weather: ☐ Sun ☐ Clouds ☐ Rain ☐ Wind ☐ Snow   Barometer:_____   Temp:____ / ____

I have felt: ☐ Cold   ☐ Hot   ☐ Comfortable   ☐ Mixed-bag   ☐ _____

TODAY'S FOOD & DRINK

Time	Food	How I Felt After Eating

Cravings: ☐ Sweet   ☐ Salty   ☐ Spicy   ☐ Bitter   ☐ _____

Water Consumed: _____ ozs. (YOUR WEIGHT DIVIDED BY 2, EQUALS [GOAL] OUNCES TO DRINK DAILY.*)

Other Liquids Consumed & How I Felt

*HIGH ELEVATION & CHRONIC-PAIN PATIENTS, CALCULATE 1 QUART WATER PER 50 POUNDS OF WEIGHT.

BATHROOM EXPERIENCES

Bowels ☐ Constipation ☐ Diarrhea	☐ Formed ☐ Pain ____ Times	☐ Loose ☐ Pain ____ Times	☐ Cowpie ☐ Pain ____ Times	☐ Soup ☐ Pain ____ Times	☐ Odor? ☐ Painful Gas ____ Times
Urine ☐ Too Often ☐ Infrequent	☐ Clear ☐ Pain ____ Times	☐ Cloudy ☐ Pain ____ Times	☐ Light Yellow ☐ Pain ____ Times	☐ Dark Yellow ☐ Pain ____ Times	☐ Odor? ☐ Pain ____ Times

BASAL* TEMPERATURE / BLOOD-SUGAR NUMBERS / NOTES / ETC.

*The temperature that registers on an oral thermometer when it is placed under the armpit first thing in the morning before any activity.

NOTE: Your regular body temperature (TEMP) is written in the oval on the top of the left-hand side.

TEMP

TODAY'S SLEEP

Last night, I went to bed at _____

I fell asleep at _____ ☐ Dreams?

I slept   ☐ Well   ☐ Restless   ☐ Insomnia

I got up _____ times to _____

Today, I woke up at _____

I felt   ☐ Rested & ready for the day

☐ Stiff   ☐ Tired   ☐ Sick   ☐ Sore   ☐ Pain

Describe _____

TODAY'S PRESCRIPTIONS AND/OR SUPPLEMENTS*

Time	Prescription/Supplement	Time	Prescription/Supplement

*NOTE: WHAT YOU APPLY TO YOUR SKIN MATTERS TOO!

TODAY'S EXERCISE

Type	Time	Distance, Pounds, Repetitions, etc.
Walking		
Running		
Cycling		
Stretching		

TODAY'S ACCOMPLISHMENTS (NO MATTER HOW INSIGNIFICANT THEY MAY SEEM)

_____

_____

_____

WEIGHT	TODAY'S RECORD	DATE

Weather: ☐ Sun ☐ Clouds ☐ Rain ☐ Wind ☐ Snow   Barometer:_____   Temp:____H__/__L__

I have felt: ☐ Cold   ☐ Hot   ☐ Comfortable   ☐ Mixed-bag   ☐ _____

TODAY'S FOOD & DRINK

Time	Food	How I Felt After Eating

Cravings: ☐ Sweet   ☐ Salty   ☐ Spicy   ☐ Bitter   ☐ _____

Water Consumed: OZS. (YOUR WEIGHT DIVIDED BY 2, EQUALS [GOAL] OUNCES TO DRINK DAILY.*)

Other Liquids Consumed & How I Felt

*HIGH ELEVATION & CHRONIC-PAIN PATIENTS, CALCULATE 1 QUART WATER PER 50 POUNDS OF WEIGHT.

BATHROOM EXPERIENCES

Bowels ☐ Constipation ☐ Diarrhea	☐ Formed ☐ Pain _____ Times	☐ Loose ☐ Pain _____ Times	☐ Cowpie ☐ Pain _____ Times	☐ Soup ☐ Pain _____ Times	☐ Odor? ☐ Painful Gas _____ Times
Urine ☐ Too Often ☐ Infrequent	☐ Clear ☐ Pain _____ Times	☐ Cloudy ☐ Pain _____ Times	☐ Light Yellow ☐ Pain _____ Times	☐ Dark Yellow ☐ Pain _____ Times	☐ Odor? ☐ Pain _____ Times

BASAL* TEMPERATURE / BLOOD-SUGAR NUMBERS / NOTES / ETC.

*The temperature that registers on an oral thermometer when it is placed under the armpit first thing in the morning before any activity.

NOTE: Your regular body temperature (TEMP) is written in the oval on the top of the left-hand side.

TEMP	TODAY'S SLEEP

Last night, I went to bed at _____   Today, I woke up at _____

I fell asleep at _____ ☐ Dreams?   I felt ☐ Rested & ready for the day

I slept ☐ Well ☐ Restless ☐ Insomnia   ☐ Stiff ☐ Tired ☐ Sick ☐ Sore ☐ Pain

I got up _____ times to _____   Describe _____

TODAY'S PRESCRIPTIONS AND/OR SUPPLEMENTS*

Time	Prescription/Supplement	Time	Prescription/Supplement

*NOTE: WHAT YOU APPLY TO YOUR SKIN MATTERS TOO!

TODAY'S EXERCISE

Type	Time	Distance, Pounds, Repetitions, etc.
Walking		
Running		
Cycling		
Stretching		

TODAY'S ACCOMPLISHMENTS (NO MATTER HOW INSIGNIFICANT THEY MAY SEEM)

_____

_____

_____

| WEIGHT | TODAY'S RECORD | DATE |

Weather: ☐ Sun ☐ Clouds ☐ Rain ☐ Wind ☐ Snow   Barometer:_____   Temp:____ H / L ____

I have felt: ☐ Cold   ☐ Hot   ☐ Comfortable   ☐ Mixed-bag   ☐ _____

TODAY'S FOOD & DRINK

Time	Food	How I Felt After Eating

Cravings: ☐ Sweet   ☐ Salty   ☐ Spicy   ☐ Bitter   ☐ _____

Water Consumed: ozs. (YOUR WEIGHT DIVIDED BY 2, EQUALS [GOAL] OUNCES TO DRINK DAILY.*)

Other Liquids Consumed & How I Felt

*HIGH ELEVATION & CHRONIC-PAIN PATIENTS, CALCULATE 1 QUART WATER PER 50 POUNDS OF WEIGHT.

BATHROOM EXPERIENCES

Bowels ☐ Constipation ☐ Diarrhea	☐ Formed ☐ Pain _____ Times	☐ Loose ☐ Pain _____ Times	☐ Cowpie ☐ Pain _____ Times	☐ Soup ☐ Pain _____ Times	☐ Odor? ☐ Painful Gas _____ Times
Urine ☐ Too Often ☐ Infrequent	☐ Clear ☐ Pain _____ Times	☐ Cloudy ☐ Pain _____ Times	☐ Light Yellow ☐ Pain _____ Times	☐ Dark Yellow ☐ Pain _____ Times	☐ Odor? ☐ Pain _____ Times

BASAL* TEMPERATURE / BLOOD-SUGAR NUMBERS / NOTES / ETC.

*The temperature that registers on an oral thermometer when it is placed under the armpit first thing in the morning before any activity.

NOTE: Your regular body temperature (TEMP) is written in the oval on the top of the left-hand side.

TEMP

TODAY'S SLEEP

Last night, I went to bed at _____

I fell asleep at _____ ☐ Dreams?

I slept ☐ Well ☐ Restless ☐ Insomnia

I got up _____ times to _____

Today, I woke up at _____

I felt ☐ Rested & ready for the day

☐ Stiff ☐ Tired ☐ Sick ☐ Sore ☐ Pain

Describe _____

TODAY'S PRESCRIPTIONS AND/OR SUPPLEMENTS*

Time	Prescription/Supplement	Time	Prescription/Supplement

*NOTE: WHAT YOU APPLY TO YOUR SKIN MATTERS TOO!

TODAY'S EXERCISE

Type	Time	Distance, Pounds, Repetitions, etc.
Walking		
Running		
Cycling		
Stretching		

TODAY'S ACCOMPLISHMENTS (NO MATTER HOW INSIGNIFICANT THEY MAY SEEM)

_____

_____

_____

TODAY'S RECORD

WEIGHT | **DATE**

Weather: ☐ Sun ☐ Clouds ☐ Rain ☐ Wind ☐ Snow   Barometer: _____   Temp: __H__ / __L__

I have felt: ☐ Cold   ☐ Hot   ☐ Comfortable   ☐ Mixed-bag   ☐ _____

TODAY'S FOOD & DRINK

Time	Food	How I Felt After Eating

Cravings: ☐ Sweet   ☐ Salty   ☐ Spicy   ☐ Bitter   ☐ _____

Water Consumed: ____ OZS. (YOUR WEIGHT DIVIDED BY 2, EQUALS [GOAL] OUNCES TO DRINK DAILY.*)

Other Liquids Consumed & How I Felt

*HIGH ELEVATION & CHRONIC-PAIN PATIENTS, CALCULATE 1 QUART WATER PER 50 POUNDS OF WEIGHT.

BATHROOM EXPERIENCES

Bowels ☐ Constipation ☐ Diarrhea	☐ Formed ☐ Pain _____ Times	☐ Loose ☐ Pain _____ Times	☐ Cowpie ☐ Pain _____ Times	☐ Soup ☐ Pain _____ Times	☐ Odor? ☐ Painful Gas _____ Times
Urine ☐ Too Often ☐ Infrequent	☐ Clear ☐ Pain _____ Times	☐ Cloudy ☐ Pain _____ Times	☐ Light Yellow ☐ Pain _____ Times	☐ Dark Yellow ☐ Pain _____ Times	☐ Odor? ☐ Pain _____ Times

BASAL* TEMPERATURE / BLOOD-SUGAR NUMBERS / NOTES / ETC.

*The temperature that registers on an oral thermometer when it is placed under the armpit first thing in the morning before any activity.

NOTE: Your regular body temperature (TEMP) is written in the oval on the top of the left-hand side.

TEMP	**TODAY'S SLEEP**

Last night, I went to bed at _____   Today, I woke up at _____

I fell asleep at _____ ☐ Dreams?   I felt ☐ Rested & ready for the day

I slept ☐ Well ☐ Restless ☐ Insomnia   ☐ Stiff ☐ Tired ☐ Sick ☐ Sore ☐ Pain

I got up _____ times to _____   Describe _____

TODAY'S PRESCRIPTIONS AND/OR SUPPLEMENTS*

Time	Prescription/Supplement	Time	Prescription/Supplement

*NOTE: WHAT YOU APPLY TO YOUR SKIN MATTERS TOO!

TODAY'S EXERCISE

Type	Time	Distance, Pounds, Repetitions, etc.
Walking		
Running		
Cycling		
Stretching		

TODAY'S ACCOMPLISHMENTS (NO MATTER HOW INSIGNIFICANT THEY MAY SEEM)

_____

_____

_____

| WEIGHT | TODAY'S RECORD | DATE |

Weather: ☐ Sun ☐ Clouds ☐ Rain ☐ Wind ☐ Snow   Barometer:_____   Temp:____ H ____ L

I have felt: ☐ Cold   ☐ Hot   ☐ Comfortable   ☐ Mixed-bag   ☐ _____

TODAY'S FOOD & DRINK

Time	Food	How I Felt After Eating

Cravings: ☐ Sweet   ☐ Salty   ☐ Spicy   ☐ Bitter   ☐ _____

Water Consumed: _____ ozs. (YOUR WEIGHT DIVIDED BY 2, EQUALS [GOAL] OUNCES TO DRINK DAILY.*)

Other Liquids Consumed & How I Felt

*HIGH ELEVATION & CHRONIC-PAIN PATIENTS, CALCULATE 1 QUART WATER PER 50 POUNDS OF WEIGHT.

BATHROOM EXPERIENCES

Bowels ☐ Constipation ☐ Diarrhea	☐ Formed ☐ Pain _____ Times	☐ Loose ☐ Pain _____ Times	☐ Cowpie ☐ Pain _____ Times	☐ Soup ☐ Pain _____ Times	☐ Odor? ☐ Painful Gas _____ Times
Urine ☐ Too Often ☐ Infrequent	☐ Clear ☐ Pain _____ Times	☐ Cloudy ☐ Pain _____ Times	☐ Light Yellow ☐ Pain _____ Times	☐ Dark Yellow ☐ Pain _____ Times	☐ Odor? ☐ Pain _____ Times

BASAL* TEMPERATURE / BLOOD-SUGAR NUMBERS / NOTES / ETC.

*The temperature that registers on an oral thermometer when it is placed under the armpit first thing in the morning before any activity.

NOTE: Your regular body temperature (TEMP) is written in the oval on the top of the left-hand side.

TEMP

TODAY'S SLEEP

Last night, I went to bed at _____

I fell asleep at _____ ☐ Dreams?

I slept ☐ Well ☐ Restless ☐ Insomnia

I got up _____ times to _____

Today, I woke up at _____

I felt ☐ Rested & ready for the day

☐ Stiff ☐ Tired ☐ Sick ☐ Sore ☐ Pain

Describe _____

TODAY'S PRESCRIPTIONS AND/OR SUPPLEMENTS*

Time	Prescription/Supplement	Time	Prescription/Supplement

*NOTE: WHAT YOU APPLY TO YOUR SKIN MATTERS TOO!

TODAY'S EXERCISE

Type	Time	Distance, Pounds, Repetitions, etc.
Walking		
Running		
Cycling		
Stretching		

TODAY'S ACCOMPLISHMENTS (NO MATTER HOW INSIGNIFICANT THEY MAY SEEM)

_____

_____

_____

WEIGHT	TODAY'S RECORD	DATE

Weather: ☐ Sun ☐ Clouds ☐ Rain ☐ Wind ☐ Snow   Barometer:_____   Temp: H___ / L___

I have felt: ☐ Cold   ☐ Hot   ☐ Comfortable   ☐ Mixed-bag   ☐ _____

TODAY'S FOOD & DRINK

Time	Food	How I Felt After Eating

Cravings: ☐ Sweet   ☐ Salty   ☐ Spicy   ☐ Bitter   ☐ _____

Water Consumed: _____ ozs. (YOUR WEIGHT DIVIDED BY 2, EQUALS [GOAL] OUNCES TO DRINK DAILY.*)

Other Liquids Consumed & How I Felt

*HIGH ELEVATION & CHRONIC-PAIN PATIENTS, CALCULATE 1 QUART WATER PER 50 POUNDS OF WEIGHT.

BATHROOM EXPERIENCES

Bowels ☐ Constipation ☐ Diarrhea	☐ Formed ☐ Pain _____ Times	☐ Loose ☐ Pain _____ Times	☐ Cowpie ☐ Pain _____ Times	☐ Soup ☐ Pain _____ Times	☐ Odor? ☐ Painful Gas _____ Times
Urine ☐ Too Often ☐ Infrequent	☐ Clear ☐ Pain _____ Times	☐ Cloudy ☐ Pain _____ Times	☐ Light Yellow ☐ Pain _____ Times	☐ Dark Yellow ☐ Pain _____ Times	☐ Odor? ☐ Pain _____ Times

BASAL* TEMPERATURE / BLOOD-SUGAR NUMBERS / NOTES / ETC.

*The temperature that registers on an oral thermometer when it is placed under the armpit first thing in the morning before any activity.

NOTE: Your regular body temperature (TEMP) is written in the oval on the top of the left-hand side.

| TEMP | **TODAY'S SLEEP** |

Last night, I went to bed at _____   Today, I woke up at _____

I fell asleep at _____ ☐ Dreams?   I felt   ☐ Rested & ready for the day

I slept ☐ Well   ☐ Restless   ☐ Insomnia   ☐ Stiff   ☐ Tired   ☐ Sick   ☐ Sore   ☐ Pain

I got up _____ times to _____   Describe _____

TODAY'S PRESCRIPTIONS AND/OR SUPPLEMENTS*

Time	Prescription/Supplement	Time	Prescription/Supplement

*NOTE: WHAT YOU APPLY TO YOUR SKIN MATTERS TOO!

TODAY'S EXERCISE

Type	Time	Distance, Pounds, Repetitions, etc.
Walking		
Running		
Cycling		
Stretching		

TODAY'S ACCOMPLISHMENTS (NO MATTER HOW INSIGNIFICANT THEY MAY SEEM)

_____

_____

_____

| WEIGHT | TODAY'S RECORD | DATE |

Weather: ☐ Sun ☐ Clouds ☐ Rain ☐ Wind ☐ Snow   Barometer:_____   Temp: H___/L___

I have felt: ☐ Cold ☐ Hot ☐ Comfortable ☐ Mixed-bag ☐ _____

TODAY'S FOOD & DRINK

Time	Food	How I Felt After Eating

Cravings: ☐ Sweet ☐ Salty ☐ Spicy ☐ Bitter ☐ _____

Water Consumed: _____ OZS. (YOUR WEIGHT DIVIDED BY 2, EQUALS [GOAL] OUNCES TO DRINK DAILY.*)

Other Liquids Consumed & How I Felt

*HIGH ELEVATION & CHRONIC-PAIN PATIENTS, CALCULATE 1 QUART WATER PER 50 POUNDS OF WEIGHT.

BATHROOM EXPERIENCES

Bowels ☐ Constipation ☐ Diarrhea	☐ Formed ☐ Pain _____ Times	☐ Loose ☐ Pain _____ Times	☐ Cowpie ☐ Pain _____ Times	☐ Soup ☐ Pain _____ Times	☐ Odor? ☐ Painful Gas _____ Times
Urine ☐ Too Often ☐ Infrequent	☐ Clear ☐ Pain _____ Times	☐ Cloudy ☐ Pain _____ Times	☐ Light Yellow ☐ Pain _____ Times	☐ Dark Yellow ☐ Pain _____ Times	☐ Odor? ☐ Pain _____ Times

BASAL* TEMPERATURE / BLOOD-SUGAR NUMBERS / NOTES / ETC.

*The temperature that registers on an oral thermometer when it is placed under the armpit first thing in the morning before any activity.

NOTE: Your regular body temperature (TEMP) is written in the oval on the top of the left-hand side.

(TEMP)

TODAY'S SLEEP

Last night, I went to bed at _____

I fell asleep at _____ ☐ Dreams?

I slept ☐ Well ☐ Restless ☐ Insomnia

I got up _____ times to _____

Today, I woke up at _____

I felt ☐ Rested & ready for the day

☐ Stiff ☐ Tired ☐ Sick ☐ Sore ☐ Pain

Describe _____

TODAY'S PRESCRIPTIONS AND/OR SUPPLEMENTS*

Time	Prescription/Supplement	Time	Prescription/Supplement

*NOTE: WHAT YOU APPLY TO YOUR SKIN MATTERS TOO!

TODAY'S EXERCISE

Type	Time	Distance, Pounds, Repetitions, etc.
Walking		
Running		
Cycling		
Stretching		

TODAY'S ACCOMPLISHMENTS (NO MATTER HOW INSIGNIFICANT THEY MAY SEEM)

_____

_____

_____

WEIGHT	TODAY'S RECORD	DATE

Weather: ☐ Sun ☐ Clouds ☐ Rain ☐ Wind ☐ Snow   Barometer:_____   Temp:____ H / L

I have felt: ☐ Cold   ☐ Hot   ☐ Comfortable   ☐ Mixed-bag   ☐ _____

TODAY'S FOOD & DRINK

Time	Food	How I Felt After Eating

Cravings: ☐ Sweet   ☐ Salty   ☐ Spicy   ☐ Bitter   ☐ _____

Water Consumed: OZS. (YOUR WEIGHT DIVIDED BY 2, EQUALS [GOAL] OUNCES TO DRINK DAILY.*)

Other Liquids Consumed & How I Felt

*HIGH ELEVATION & CHRONIC-PAIN PATIENTS, CALCULATE 1 QUART WATER PER 50 POUNDS OF WEIGHT.

BATHROOM EXPERIENCES

Bowels ☐ Constipation ☐ Diarrhea	☐ Formed ☐ Pain _____ Times	☐ Loose ☐ Pain _____ Times	☐ Cowpie ☐ Pain _____ Times	☐ Soup ☐ Pain _____ Times	☐ Odor? ☐ Painful Gas _____ Times
Urine ☐ Too Often ☐ Infrequent	☐ Clear ☐ Pain _____ Times	☐ Cloudy ☐ Pain _____ Times	☐ Light Yellow ☐ Pain _____ Times	☐ Dark Yellow ☐ Pain _____ Times	☐ Odor? ☐ Pain _____ Times

BASAL* TEMPERATURE / BLOOD-SUGAR NUMBERS / NOTES / ETC.

*The temperature that registers on an oral thermometer when it is placed under the armpit first thing in the morning before any activity.

NOTE: Your regular body temperature (TEMP) is written in the oval on the top of the left-hand side.

(TEMP)

TODAY'S SLEEP

Last night, I went to bed at _____

I fell asleep at _____ ☐ Dreams?

I slept ☐ Well ☐ Restless ☐ Insomnia

I got up _____ times to _____

Today, I woke up at _____

I felt ☐ Rested & ready for the day

☐ Stiff ☐ Tired ☐ Sick ☐ Sore ☐ Pain

Describe _____

TODAY'S PRESCRIPTIONS AND/OR SUPPLEMENTS*

Time	Prescription/Supplement	Time	Prescription/Supplement

*NOTE: WHAT YOU APPLY TO YOUR SKIN MATTERS TOO!

TODAY'S EXERCISE

Type	Time	Distance, Pounds, Repetitions, etc.
Walking		
Running		
Cycling		
Stretching		

TODAY'S ACCOMPLISHMENTS (NO MATTER HOW INSIGNIFICANT THEY MAY SEEM)

_____

_____

_____

WEIGHT | TODAY'S RECORD | DATE

Weather: ☐ Sun ☐ Clouds ☐ Rain ☐ Wind ☐ Snow   Barometer:_____   Temp:____ ____

I have felt: ☐ Cold   ☐ Hot   ☐ Comfortable   ☐ Mixed-bag   ☐ _____

TODAY'S FOOD & DRINK

Time	Food	How I Felt After Eating

Cravings: ☐ Sweet   ☐ Salty   ☐ Spicy   ☐ Bitter   ☐ _____

Water Consumed: _____ ozs. (YOUR WEIGHT DIVIDED BY 2, EQUALS [GOAL] OUNCES TO DRINK DAILY.*)

Other Liquids Consumed & How I Felt

*HIGH ELEVATION & CHRONIC-PAIN PATIENTS, CALCULATE 1 QUART WATER PER 50 POUNDS OF WEIGHT.

BATHROOM EXPERIENCES

Bowels ☐ Constipation ☐ Diarrhea	☐ Formed ☐ Pain _____ Times	☐ Loose ☐ Pain _____ Times	☐ Cowpie ☐ Pain _____ Times	☐ Soup ☐ Pain _____ Times	☐ Odor? ☐ Painful Gas _____ Times
Urine ☐ Too Often ☐ Infrequent	☐ Clear ☐ Pain _____ Times	☐ Cloudy ☐ Pain _____ Times	☐ Light Yellow ☐ Pain _____ Times	☐ Dark Yellow ☐ Pain _____ Times	☐ Odor? ☐ Pain _____ Times

BASAL* TEMPERATURE / BLOOD-SUGAR NUMBERS / NOTES / ETC.

*The temperature that registers on an oral thermometer when it is placed under the armpit first thing in the morning before any activity.

NOTE: Your regular body temperature (TEMP) is written in the oval on the top of the left-hand side.

TEMP

TODAY'S SLEEP

Last night, I went to bed at _____

I fell asleep at _____ ☐ Dreams?

I slept ☐ Well   ☐ Restless   ☐ Insomnia

I got up _____ times to _____

Today, I woke up at _____

I felt   ☐ Rested & ready for the day

☐ Stiff   ☐ Tired   ☐ Sick   ☐ Sore   ☐ Pain

Describe _____

TODAY'S PRESCRIPTIONS AND/OR SUPPLEMENTS*

Time	Prescription/Supplement	Time	Prescription/Supplement

*NOTE: WHAT YOU APPLY TO YOUR SKIN MATTERS TOO!

TODAY'S EXERCISE

Type	Time	Distance, Pounds, Repetitions, etc.
Walking		
Running		
Cycling		
Stretching		

TODAY'S ACCOMPLISHMENTS (NO MATTER HOW INSIGNIFICANT THEY MAY SEEM)

_____

_____

_____

WEIGHT	TODAY'S RECORD	DATE

Weather: ☐ Sun ☐ Clouds ☐ Rain ☐ Wind ☐ Snow   Barometer:_____   Temp:____ H / L____

I have felt: ☐ Cold   ☐ Hot   ☐ Comfortable   ☐ Mixed-bag   ☐ _____

TODAY'S FOOD & DRINK

Time	Food	How I Felt After Eating

Cravings: ☐ Sweet   ☐ Salty   ☐ Spicy   ☐ Bitter   ☐ _____

Water Consumed: _____ OZS. (YOUR WEIGHT DIVIDED BY 2, EQUALS [GOAL] OUNCES TO DRINK DAILY.*)

Other Liquids Consumed & How I Felt

*HIGH ELEVATION & CHRONIC-PAIN PATIENTS, CALCULATE 1 QUART WATER PER 50 POUNDS OF WEIGHT.

BATHROOM EXPERIENCES

Bowels ☐ Constipation ☐ Diarrhea	☐ Formed ☐ Pain _____ Times	☐ Loose ☐ Pain _____ Times	☐ Cowpie ☐ Pain _____ Times	☐ Soup ☐ Pain _____ Times	☐ Odor? ☐ Painful Gas _____ Times
Urine ☐ Too Often ☐ Infrequent	☐ Clear ☐ Pain _____ Times	☐ Cloudy ☐ Pain _____ Times	☐ Light Yellow ☐ Pain _____ Times	☐ Dark Yellow ☐ Pain _____ Times	☐ Odor? ☐ Pain _____ Times

BASAL* TEMPERATURE / BLOOD-SUGAR NUMBERS / NOTES / ETC.

*The temperature that registers on an oral thermometer when it is placed under the armpit first thing in the morning before any activity.

NOTE: Your regular body temperature (TEMP) is written in the oval on the top of the left-hand side.

TEMP | TODAY'S SLEEP

Last night, I went to bed at _____   Today, I woke up at _____

I fell asleep at _____ ☐ Dreams?   I felt ☐ Rested & ready for the day

I slept ☐ Well ☐ Restless ☐ Insomnia   ☐ Stiff ☐ Tired ☐ Sick ☐ Sore ☐ Pain

I got up _____ times to _____   Describe _____

TODAY'S PRESCRIPTIONS AND/OR SUPPLEMENTS*

Time	Prescription/Supplement	Time	Prescription/Supplement

*NOTE: WHAT YOU APPLY TO YOUR SKIN MATTERS TOO!

TODAY'S EXERCISE

Type	Time	Distance, Pounds, Repetitions, etc.
Walking		
Running		
Cycling		
Stretching		

TODAY'S ACCOMPLISHMENTS (NO MATTER HOW INSIGNIFICANT THEY MAY SEEM)

_____

_____

_____

| WEIGHT | TODAY'S RECORD | DATE |

Weather: ☐ Sun ☐ Clouds ☐ Rain ☐ Wind ☐ Snow   Barometer:_____   Temp:_____

I have felt: ☐ Cold   ☐ Hot   ☐ Comfortable   ☐ Mixed-bag   ☐ _____

TODAY'S FOOD & DRINK

Time	Food	How I Felt After Eating

Cravings: ☐ Sweet   ☐ Salty   ☐ Spicy   ☐ Bitter   ☐ _____

Water Consumed: ozs. (YOUR WEIGHT DIVIDED BY 2, EQUALS [GOAL] OUNCES TO DRINK DAILY.*)

Other Liquids Consumed & How I Felt

*HIGH ELEVATION & CHRONIC-PAIN PATIENTS, CALCULATE 1 QUART WATER PER 50 POUNDS OF WEIGHT.

BATHROOM EXPERIENCES

Bowels ☐ Constipation ☐ Diarrhea	☐ Formed ☐ Pain _____ Times	☐ Loose ☐ Pain _____ Times	☐ Cowpie ☐ Pain _____ Times	☐ Soup ☐ Pain _____ Times	☐ Odor? ☐ Painful Gas _____ Times
Urine ☐ Too Often ☐ Infrequent	☐ Clear ☐ Pain _____ Times	☐ Cloudy ☐ Pain _____ Times	☐ Light Yellow ☐ Pain _____ Times	☐ Dark Yellow ☐ Pain _____ Times	☐ Odor? ☐ Pain _____ Times

BASAL* TEMPERATURE / BLOOD-SUGAR NUMBERS / NOTES / ETC.

*The temperature that registers on an oral thermometer when it is placed under the armpit first thing in the morning before any activity.

NOTE: Your regular body temperature (TEMP) is written in the oval on the top of the left-hand side.

TEMP

TODAY'S SLEEP

Last night, I went to bed at _____

I fell asleep at _____ ☐ Dreams?

I slept ☐ Well ☐ Restless ☐ Insomnia

I got up _____ times to _____

Today, I woke up at _____

I felt ☐ Rested & ready for the day

☐ Stiff ☐ Tired ☐ Sick ☐ Sore ☐ Pain

Describe _____

TODAY'S PRESCRIPTIONS AND/OR SUPPLEMENTS*

Time	Prescription/Supplement	Time	Prescription/Supplement

*NOTE: WHAT YOU APPLY TO YOUR SKIN MATTERS TOO!

TODAY'S EXERCISE

Type	Time	Distance, Pounds, Repetitions, etc.
Walking		
Running		
Cycling		
Stretching		

TODAY'S ACCOMPLISHMENTS (NO MATTER HOW INSIGNIFICANT THEY MAY SEEM)

_____

_____

_____

| WEIGHT | TODAY'S RECORD | DATE |

Weather: ☐ Sun ☐ Clouds ☐ Rain ☐ Wind ☐ Snow   Barometer:_____   Temp:____H_/_L_

I have felt: ☐ Cold   ☐ Hot   ☐ Comfortable   ☐ Mixed-bag   ☐ _____

TODAY'S FOOD & DRINK

Time	Food	How I Felt After Eating

Cravings: ☐ Sweet   ☐ Salty   ☐ Spicy   ☐ Bitter   ☐ _____

Water Consumed: OZS. (YOUR WEIGHT DIVIDED BY 2, EQUALS [GOAL] OUNCES TO DRINK DAILY.*)

Other Liquids Consumed & How I Felt

*HIGH ELEVATION & CHRONIC-PAIN PATIENTS, CALCULATE 1 QUART WATER PER 50 POUNDS OF WEIGHT.

BATHROOM EXPERIENCES

Bowels ☐ Constipation ☐ Diarrhea	☐ Formed ☐ Pain _____ Times	☐ Loose ☐ Pain _____ Times	☐ Cowpie ☐ Pain _____ Times	☐ Soup ☐ Pain _____ Times	☐ Odor? ☐ Painful Gas _____ Times
Urine ☐ Too Often ☐ Infrequent	☐ Clear ☐ Pain _____ Times	☐ Cloudy ☐ Pain _____ Times	☐ Light Yellow ☐ Pain _____ Times	☐ Dark Yellow ☐ Pain _____ Times	☐ Odor? ☐ Pain _____ Times

BASAL* TEMPERATURE / BLOOD-SUGAR NUMBERS / NOTES / ETC.

*The temperature that registers on an oral thermometer when it is placed under the armpit first thing in the morning before any activity.

NOTE: Your regular body temperature (TEMP) is written in the oval on the top of the left-hand side.

TEMP	TODAY'S SLEEP

Last night, I went to bed at _____   Today, I woke up at _____

I fell asleep at _____ ☐ Dreams?   I felt ☐ Rested & ready for the day

I slept ☐ Well ☐ Restless ☐ Insomnia   ☐ Stiff ☐ Tired ☐ Sick ☐ Sore ☐ Pain

I got up _____ times to _____   Describe _____

TODAY'S PRESCRIPTIONS AND/OR SUPPLEMENTS*

Time	Prescription/Supplement	Time	Prescription/Supplement

*NOTE: WHAT YOU APPLY TO YOUR SKIN MATTERS TOO!

TODAY'S EXERCISE

Type	Time	Distance, Pounds, Repetitions, etc.
Walking		
Running		
Cycling		
Stretching		

TODAY'S ACCOMPLISHMENTS (NO MATTER HOW INSIGNIFICANT THEY MAY SEEM)

_____

_____

_____

WEIGHT	TODAY'S RECORD	DATE

Weather: ☐ Sun ☐ Clouds ☐ Rain ☐ Wind ☐ Snow   Barometer: _____   Temp: ____ H / L

I have felt: ☐ Cold   ☐ Hot   ☐ Comfortable   ☐ Mixed-bag   ☐ _____

TODAY'S FOOD & DRINK

Time	Food	How I Felt After Eating

Cravings: ☐ Sweet   ☐ Salty   ☐ Spicy   ☐ Bitter   ☐ _____

Water Consumed: _____ ozs. (YOUR WEIGHT DIVIDED BY 2, EQUALS [GOAL] OUNCES TO DRINK DAILY.*)

Other Liquids Consumed & How I Felt

*HIGH ELEVATION & CHRONIC-PAIN PATIENTS, CALCULATE 1 QUART WATER PER 50 POUNDS OF WEIGHT.

BATHROOM EXPERIENCES

Bowels ☐ Constipation ☐ Diarrhea	☐ Formed ☐ Pain _____ Times	☐ Loose ☐ Pain _____ Times	☐ Cowpie ☐ Pain _____ Times	☐ Soup ☐ Pain _____ Times	☐ Odor? ☐ Painful Gas _____ Times
Urine ☐ Too Often ☐ Infrequent	☐ Clear ☐ Pain _____ Times	☐ Cloudy ☐ Pain _____ Times	☐ Light Yellow ☐ Pain _____ Times	☐ Dark Yellow ☐ Pain _____ Times	☐ Odor? ☐ Pain _____ Times

BASAL* TEMPERATURE / BLOOD-SUGAR NUMBERS / NOTES / ETC.

*The temperature that registers on an oral thermometer when it is placed under the armpit first thing in the morning before any activity.

NOTE: Your regular body temperature (TEMP) is written in the oval on the top of the left-hand side.

TEMP

TODAY'S SLEEP

Last night, I went to bed at _____

I fell asleep at _____ ☐ Dreams?

I slept ☐ Well ☐ Restless ☐ Insomnia

I got up _____ times to _____

Today, I woke up at _____

I felt ☐ Rested & ready for the day

☐ Stiff ☐ Tired ☐ Sick ☐ Sore ☐ Pain

Describe _____

TODAY'S PRESCRIPTIONS AND/OR SUPPLEMENTS*

Time	Prescription/Supplement	Time	Prescription/Supplement

*NOTE: WHAT YOU APPLY TO YOUR SKIN MATTERS TOO!

TODAY'S EXERCISE

Type	Time	Distance, Pounds, Repetitions, etc.
Walking		
Running		
Cycling		
Stretching		

TODAY'S ACCOMPLISHMENTS (NO MATTER HOW INSIGNIFICANT THEY MAY SEEM)

_____

_____

_____

| WEIGHT | TODAY'S RECORD | DATE |

Weather: ☐ Sun ☐ Clouds ☐ Rain ☐ Wind ☐ Snow   Barometer:_____   Temp:__H__/__L__

I have felt: ☐ Cold   ☐ Hot   ☐ Comfortable   ☐ Mixed-bag   ☐ _____

TODAY'S FOOD & DRINK

Time	Food	How I Felt After Eating

Cravings: ☐ Sweet   ☐ Salty   ☐ Spicy   ☐ Bitter   ☐ _____

Water Consumed: _____ ozs. (YOUR WEIGHT DIVIDED BY 2, EQUALS [GOAL] OUNCES TO DRINK DAILY.*)

Other Liquids Consumed & How I Felt

*HIGH ELEVATION & CHRONIC-PAIN PATIENTS, CALCULATE 1 QUART WATER PER 50 POUNDS OF WEIGHT.

BATHROOM EXPERIENCES

Bowels ☐ Constipation ☐ Diarrhea	☐ Formed ☐ Pain ____ Times	☐ Loose ☐ Pain ____ Times	☐ Cowpie ☐ Pain ____ Times	☐ Soup ☐ Pain ____ Times	☐ Odor? ☐ Painful Gas ____ Times
Urine ☐ Too Often ☐ Infrequent	☐ Clear ☐ Pain ____ Times	☐ Cloudy ☐ Pain ____ Times	☐ Light Yellow ☐ Pain ____ Times	☐ Dark Yellow ☐ Pain ____ Times	☐ Odor? ☐ Pain ____ Times

BASAL* TEMPERATURE / BLOOD-SUGAR NUMBERS / NOTES / ETC.

*The temperature that registers on an oral thermometer when it is placed under the armpit first thing in the morning before any activity.

NOTE: Your regular body temperature (TEMP) is written in the oval on the top of the left-hand side.

| TEMP | **TODAY'S SLEEP** |

Last night, I went to bed at _____   Today, I woke up at _____

I fell asleep at _____ ☐ Dreams?   I felt   ☐ Rested & ready for the day

I slept   ☐ Well   ☐ Restless   ☐ Insomnia   ☐ Stiff   ☐ Tired   ☐ Sick   ☐ Sore   ☐ Pain

I got up _____ times to _____   Describe _____

TODAY'S PRESCRIPTIONS AND/OR SUPPLEMENTS*

Time	Prescription/Supplement	Time	Prescription/Supplement

*NOTE: WHAT YOU APPLY TO YOUR SKIN MATTERS TOO!

TODAY'S EXERCISE

Type	Time	Distance, Pounds, Repetitions, etc.
Walking		
Running		
Cycling		
Stretching		

TODAY'S ACCOMPLISHMENTS (NO MATTER HOW INSIGNIFICANT THEY MAY SEEM)

_____

_____

_____

| WEIGHT | TODAY'S RECORD | DATE |

Weather: ☐ Sun ☐ Clouds ☐ Rain ☐ Wind ☐ Snow   Barometer:_____   Temp:____ H / L

I have felt: ☐ Cold ☐ Hot ☐ Comfortable ☐ Mixed-bag ☐ _____

TODAY'S FOOD & DRINK

Time	Food	How I Felt After Eating

Cravings: ☐ Sweet ☐ Salty ☐ Spicy ☐ Bitter ☐ _____

Water Consumed: ____ ozs. (YOUR WEIGHT DIVIDED BY 2, EQUALS [GOAL] OUNCES TO DRINK DAILY.*)

Other Liquids Consumed & How I Felt

*HIGH ELEVATION & CHRONIC-PAIN PATIENTS, CALCULATE 1 QUART WATER PER 50 POUNDS OF WEIGHT.

BATHROOM EXPERIENCES

Bowels ☐ Constipation ☐ Diarrhea	☐ Formed ☐ Pain ____ Times	☐ Loose ☐ Pain ____ Times	☐ Cowpie ☐ Pain ____ Times	☐ Soup ☐ Pain ____ Times	☐ Odor? ☐ Painful Gas ____ Times
Urine ☐ Too Often ☐ Infrequent	☐ Clear ☐ Pain ____ Times	☐ Cloudy ☐ Pain ____ Times	☐ Light Yellow ☐ Pain ____ Times	☐ Dark Yellow ☐ Pain ____ Times	☐ Odor? ☐ Pain ____ Times

BASAL* TEMPERATURE / BLOOD-SUGAR NUMBERS / NOTES / ETC.

*The temperature that registers on an oral thermometer when it is placed under the armpit first thing in the morning before any activity.

NOTE: Your regular body temperature (TEMP) is written in the oval on the top of the left-hand side.

TEMP

TODAY'S SLEEP

Last night, I went to bed at _____

I fell asleep at _____ ☐ Dreams?

I slept ☐ Well ☐ Restless ☐ Insomnia

I got up _____ times to _____

Today, I woke up at _____

I felt ☐ Rested & ready for the day

☐ Stiff ☐ Tired ☐ Sick ☐ Sore ☐ Pain

Describe _____

TODAY'S PRESCRIPTIONS AND/OR SUPPLEMENTS*

Time	Prescription/Supplement	Time	Prescription/Supplement

*NOTE: WHAT YOU APPLY TO YOUR SKIN MATTERS TOO!

TODAY'S EXERCISE

Type	Time	Distance, Pounds, Repetitions, etc.
Walking		
Running		
Cycling		
Stretching		

TODAY'S ACCOMPLISHMENTS (NO MATTER HOW INSIGNIFICANT THEY MAY SEEM)

_____

_____

_____

| WEIGHT | **TODAY'S RECORD** | DATE |

Weather: ☐ Sun ☐ Clouds ☐ Rain ☐ Wind ☐ Snow   Barometer:_____   Temp: H__/L__

I have felt: ☐ Cold   ☐ Hot   ☐ Comfortable   ☐ Mixed-bag   ☐ _____

TODAY'S FOOD & DRINK

Time	Food	How I Felt After Eating

Cravings: ☐ Sweet   ☐ Salty   ☐ Spicy   ☐ Bitter   ☐ _____

Water Consumed: OZS.   (YOUR WEIGHT DIVIDED BY 2, EQUALS [GOAL] OUNCES TO DRINK DAILY.*)

Other Liquids Consumed & How I Felt

*HIGH ELEVATION & CHRONIC-PAIN PATIENTS, CALCULATE 1 QUART WATER PER 50 POUNDS OF WEIGHT.

BATHROOM EXPERIENCES

| **Bowels**
☐ Constipation
☐ Diarrhea | ☐ Formed
☐ Pain
____ Times | ☐ Loose
☐ Pain
____ Times | ☐ Cowpie
☐ Pain
____ Times | ☐ Soup
☐ Pain
____ Times | ☐ Odor?
☐ Painful Gas
____ Times |
| **Urine**
☐ Too Often
☐ Infrequent | ☐ Clear
☐ Pain
____ Times | ☐ Cloudy
☐ Pain
____ Times | ☐ Light Yellow
☐ Pain
____ Times | ☐ Dark Yellow
☐ Pain
____ Times | ☐ Odor?
☐ Pain
____ Times |

BASAL* TEMPERATURE / BLOOD-SUGAR NUMBERS / NOTES / ETC.

*The temperature that registers on an oral thermometer when it is placed under the armpit first thing in the morning before any activity.

NOTE: Your regular body temperature (TEMP) is written in the oval on the top of the left-hand side.

TEMP

TODAY'S SLEEP

Last night, I went to bed at _____   Today, I woke up at _____

I fell asleep at _____ ☐ Dreams?   I felt ☐ Rested & ready for the day

I slept ☐ Well ☐ Restless ☐ Insomnia   ☐ Stiff ☐ Tired ☐ Sick ☐ Sore ☐ Pain

I got up _____ times to _____   Describe _____

TODAY'S PRESCRIPTIONS AND/OR SUPPLEMENTS*

Time	Prescription/Supplement	Time	Prescription/Supplement

*NOTE: WHAT YOU APPLY TO YOUR SKIN MATTERS TOO!

TODAY'S EXERCISE

Type	Time	Distance, Pounds, Repetitions, etc.
Walking		
Running		
Cycling		
Stretching		

TODAY'S ACCOMPLISHMENTS (NO MATTER HOW INSIGNIFICANT THEY MAY SEEM)

_____

_____

_____

WEIGHT	TODAY'S RECORD	DATE

Weather: ☐ Sun ☐ Clouds ☐ Rain ☐ Wind ☐ Snow   Barometer:_____   Temp:____ /____

I have felt: ☐ Cold   ☐ Hot   ☐ Comfortable   ☐ Mixed-bag   ☐ _____

TODAY'S FOOD & DRINK

Time	Food	How I Felt After Eating

Cravings: ☐ Sweet   ☐ Salty   ☐ Spicy   ☐ Bitter   ☐ _____

Water Consumed: _____ OZS. (YOUR WEIGHT DIVIDED BY 2, EQUALS [GOAL] OUNCES TO DRINK DAILY.*)

Other Liquids Consumed & How I Felt

*HIGH ELEVATION & CHRONIC-PAIN PATIENTS, CALCULATE 1 QUART WATER PER 50 POUNDS OF WEIGHT.

BATHROOM EXPERIENCES

Bowels ☐ Constipation ☐ Diarrhea	☐ Formed ☐ Pain _____ Times	☐ Loose ☐ Pain _____ Times	☐ Cowpie ☐ Pain _____ Times	☐ Soup ☐ Pain _____ Times	☐ Odor? ☐ Painful Gas _____ Times
Urine ☐ Too Often ☐ Infrequent	☐ Clear ☐ Pain _____ Times	☐ Cloudy ☐ Pain _____ Times	☐ Light Yellow ☐ Pain _____ Times	☐ Dark Yellow ☐ Pain _____ Times	☐ Odor? ☐ Pain _____ Times

BASAL* TEMPERATURE / BLOOD-SUGAR NUMBERS / NOTES / ETC.

*The temperature that registers on an oral thermometer when it is placed under the armpit first thing in the morning before any activity.

NOTE: Your regular body temperature (TEMP) is written in the oval on the top of the left-hand side.

TEMP

TODAY'S SLEEP

Last night, I went to bed at _____

I fell asleep at _____ ☐ Dreams?

I slept ☐ Well ☐ Restless ☐ Insomnia

I got up _____ times to _____

Today, I woke up at _____

I felt ☐ Rested & ready for the day

☐ Stiff ☐ Tired ☐ Sick ☐ Sore ☐ Pain

Describe _____

TODAY'S PRESCRIPTIONS AND/OR SUPPLEMENTS*

Time	Prescription/Supplement	Time	Prescription/Supplement

*NOTE: WHAT YOU APPLY TO YOUR SKIN MATTERS TOO!

TODAY'S EXERCISE

Type	Time	Distance, Pounds, Repetitions, etc.
Walking		
Running		
Cycling		
Stretching		

TODAY'S ACCOMPLISHMENTS (NO MATTER HOW INSIGNIFICANT THEY MAY SEEM)

_____

_____

_____

| WEIGHT | TODAY'S RECORD | DATE |

Weather: ☐ Sun ☐ Clouds ☐ Rain ☐ Wind ☐ Snow   Barometer: _____   Temp: H___ / L___

I have felt: ☐ Cold ☐ Hot ☐ Comfortable ☐ Mixed-bag ☐ _____

TODAY'S FOOD & DRINK

Time	Food	How I Felt After Eating

Cravings: ☐ Sweet ☐ Salty ☐ Spicy ☐ Bitter ☐ _____

Water Consumed: OZS. (YOUR WEIGHT DIVIDED BY 2, EQUALS [GOAL] OUNCES TO DRINK DAILY.*)

Other Liquids Consumed & How I Felt

*HIGH ELEVATION & CHRONIC-PAIN PATIENTS, CALCULATE 1 QUART WATER PER 50 POUNDS OF WEIGHT.

BATHROOM EXPERIENCES

Bowels ☐ Constipation ☐ Diarrhea	☐ Formed ☐ Pain _____ Times	☐ Loose ☐ Pain _____ Times	☐ Cowpie ☐ Pain _____ Times	☐ Soup ☐ Pain _____ Times	☐ Odor? ☐ Painful Gas _____ Times
Urine ☐ Too Often ☐ Infrequent	☐ Clear ☐ Pain _____ Times	☐ Cloudy ☐ Pain _____ Times	☐ Light Yellow ☐ Pain _____ Times	☐ Dark Yellow ☐ Pain _____ Times	☐ Odor? ☐ Pain _____ Times

BASAL* TEMPERATURE / BLOOD-SUGAR NUMBERS / NOTES / ETC.

*The temperature that registers on an oral thermometer when it is placed under the armpit first thing in the morning before any activity.

NOTE: Your regular body temperature (TEMP) is written in the oval on the top of the left-hand side.

TEMP

TODAY'S SLEEP

Last night, I went to bed at _____ Today, I woke up at _____

I fell asleep at _____ ☐ Dreams? I felt ☐ Rested & ready for the day

I slept ☐ Well ☐ Restless ☐ Insomnia   ☐ Stiff ☐ Tired ☐ Sick ☐ Sore ☐ Pain

I got up _____ times to _____ Describe _____

TODAY'S PRESCRIPTIONS AND/OR SUPPLEMENTS*

Time	Prescription/Supplement	Time	Prescription/Supplement

*NOTE: WHAT YOU APPLY TO YOUR SKIN MATTERS TOO!

TODAY'S EXERCISE

Type	Time	Distance, Pounds, Repetitions, etc.
Walking		
Running		
Cycling		
Stretching		

TODAY'S ACCOMPLISHMENTS (NO MATTER HOW INSIGNIFICANT THEY MAY SEEM)

_____

_____

_____

| WEIGHT | **TODAY'S RECORD** | DATE |

Weather: ☐ Sun ☐ Clouds ☐ Rain ☐ Wind ☐ Snow   Barometer:_____   Temp:____/____

I have felt: ☐ Cold ☐ Hot ☐ Comfortable ☐ Mixed-bag ☐ _____

TODAY'S FOOD & DRINK

Time	Food	How I Felt After Eating

Cravings: ☐ Sweet ☐ Salty ☐ Spicy ☐ Bitter ☐ _____

Water Consumed: ____ ozs. (YOUR WEIGHT DIVIDED BY 2, EQUALS [GOAL] OUNCES TO DRINK DAILY.*)

Other Liquids Consumed & How I Felt

*HIGH ELEVATION & CHRONIC-PAIN PATIENTS, CALCULATE 1 QUART WATER PER 50 POUNDS OF WEIGHT.

BATHROOM EXPERIENCES

Bowels ☐ Constipation ☐ Diarrhea	☐ Formed ☐ Pain ____ Times	☐ Loose ☐ Pain ____ Times	☐ Cowpie ☐ Pain ____ Times	☐ Soup ☐ Pain ____ Times	☐ Odor? ☐ Painful Gas ____ Times
Urine ☐ Too Often ☐ Infrequent	☐ Clear ☐ Pain ____ Times	☐ Cloudy ☐ Pain ____ Times	☐ Light Yellow ☐ Pain ____ Times	☐ Dark Yellow ☐ Pain ____ Times	☐ Odor? ☐ Pain ____ Times

BASAL* TEMPERATURE / BLOOD-SUGAR NUMBERS / NOTES / ETC.

*The temperature that registers on an oral thermometer when it is placed under the armpit first thing in the morning before any activity.

NOTE: Your regular body temperature (TEMP) is written in the oval on the top of the left-hand side.

TEMP

TODAY'S SLEEP

Last night, I went to bed at _____

I fell asleep at _____ ☐ Dreams?

I slept ☐ Well ☐ Restless ☐ Insomnia

I got up _____ times to _____

Today, I woke up at _____

I felt ☐ Rested & ready for the day

☐ Stiff ☐ Tired ☐ Sick ☐ Sore ☐ Pain

Describe _____

TODAY'S PRESCRIPTIONS AND/OR SUPPLEMENTS*

Time	Prescription/Supplement	Time	Prescription/Supplement

*NOTE: WHAT YOU APPLY TO YOUR SKIN MATTERS TOO!

TODAY'S EXERCISE

Type	Time	Distance, Pounds, Repetitions, etc.
Walking		
Running		
Cycling		
Stretching		

TODAY'S ACCOMPLISHMENTS (NO MATTER HOW INSIGNIFICANT THEY MAY SEEM)

_____

_____

_____

| WEIGHT | TODAY'S RECORD | DATE |

Weather: ☐ Sun ☐ Clouds ☐ Rain ☐ Wind ☐ Snow   Barometer:_____   Temp:___H_/_L_

I have felt: ☐ Cold   ☐ Hot   ☐ Comfortable   ☐ Mixed-bag   ☐ _____

TODAY'S FOOD & DRINK

Time	Food	How I Felt After Eating

Cravings: ☐ Sweet   ☐ Salty   ☐ Spicy   ☐ Bitter   ☐ _____

Water Consumed: OZS. (YOUR WEIGHT DIVIDED BY 2, EQUALS [GOAL] OUNCES TO DRINK DAILY.*)

Other Liquids Consumed & How I Felt

*HIGH ELEVATION & CHRONIC-PAIN PATIENTS, CALCULATE 1 QUART WATER PER 50 POUNDS OF WEIGHT.

BATHROOM EXPERIENCES

Bowels ☐ Constipation ☐ Diarrhea	☐ Formed ☐ Pain _____ Times	☐ Loose ☐ Pain _____ Times	☐ Cowpie ☐ Pain _____ Times	☐ Soup ☐ Pain _____ Times	☐ Odor? ☐ Painful Gas _____ Times
Urine ☐ Too Often ☐ Infrequent	☐ Clear ☐ Pain _____ Times	☐ Cloudy ☐ Pain _____ Times	☐ Light Yellow ☐ Pain _____ Times	☐ Dark Yellow ☐ Pain _____ Times	☐ Odor? ☐ Pain _____ Times

BASAL* TEMPERATURE / BLOOD-SUGAR NUMBERS / NOTES / ETC.

*The temperature that registers on an oral thermometer when it is placed under the armpit first thing in the morning before any activity.

NOTE: Your regular body temperature (TEMP) is written in the oval on the top of the left-hand side.

(TEMP)

TODAY'S SLEEP

Last night, I went to bed at _____   Today, I woke up at _____

I fell asleep at _____ ☐ Dreams?   I felt   ☐ Rested & ready for the day

I slept ☐ Well ☐ Restless ☐ Insomnia   ☐ Stiff ☐ Tired ☐ Sick ☐ Sore ☐ Pain

I got up _____ times to _____   Describe _____

TODAY'S PRESCRIPTIONS AND/OR SUPPLEMENTS*

Time	Prescription/Supplement	Time	Prescription/Supplement

*NOTE: WHAT YOU APPLY TO YOUR SKIN MATTERS TOO!

TODAY'S EXERCISE

Type	Time	Distance, Pounds, Repetitions, etc.
Walking		
Running		
Cycling		
Stretching		

TODAY'S ACCOMPLISHMENTS (NO MATTER HOW INSIGNIFICANT THEY MAY SEEM)

_____

_____

_____

| WEIGHT | TODAY'S RECORD | DATE |

Weather: ☐ Sun ☐ Clouds ☐ Rain ☐ Wind ☐ Snow   Barometer:_____   Temp:____ ____

I have felt: ☐ Cold ☐ Hot ☐ Comfortable ☐ Mixed-bag ☐ _____

TODAY'S FOOD & DRINK

Time	Food	How I Felt After Eating

Cravings: ☐ Sweet   ☐ Salty   ☐ Spicy   ☐ Bitter   ☐ _____

Water Consumed: _____ ozs. (YOUR WEIGHT DIVIDED BY 2, EQUALS [GOAL] OUNCES TO DRINK DAILY.*)

Other Liquids Consumed & How I Felt

*HIGH ELEVATION & CHRONIC-PAIN PATIENTS, CALCULATE 1 QUART WATER PER 50 POUNDS OF WEIGHT.

BATHROOM EXPERIENCES

Bowels ☐ Constipation ☐ Diarrhea	☐ Formed ☐ Pain _____ Times	☐ Loose ☐ Pain _____ Times	☐ Cowpie ☐ Pain _____ Times	☐ Soup ☐ Pain _____ Times	☐ Odor? ☐ Painful Gas _____ Times
Urine ☐ Too Often ☐ Infrequent	☐ Clear ☐ Pain _____ Times	☐ Cloudy ☐ Pain _____ Times	☐ Light Yellow ☐ Pain _____ Times	☐ Dark Yellow ☐ Pain _____ Times	☐ Odor? ☐ Pain _____ Times

BASAL* TEMPERATURE / BLOOD-SUGAR NUMBERS / NOTES / ETC.

*The temperature that registers on an oral thermometer when it is placed under the armpit first thing in the morning before any activity.

NOTE: Your regular body temperature (TEMP) is written in the oval on the top of the left-hand side.

TEMP

TODAY'S SLEEP

Last night, I went to bed at _____

I fell asleep at _____ ☐ Dreams?

I slept ☐ Well ☐ Restless ☐ Insomnia

I got up _____ times to _____

Today, I woke up at _____

I felt ☐ Rested & ready for the day

☐ Stiff ☐ Tired ☐ Sick ☐ Sore ☐ Pain

Describe _____

TODAY'S PRESCRIPTIONS AND/OR SUPPLEMENTS*

Time	Prescription/Supplement	Time	Prescription/Supplement

*NOTE: WHAT YOU APPLY TO YOUR SKIN MATTERS TOO!

TODAY'S EXERCISE

Type	Time	Distance, Pounds, Repetitions, etc.
Walking		
Running		
Cycling		
Stretching		

TODAY'S ACCOMPLISHMENTS (NO MATTER HOW INSIGNIFICANT THEY MAY SEEM)

_____

_____

_____

| WEIGHT | TODAY'S RECORD | DATE |

Weather: ☐ Sun ☐ Clouds ☐ Rain ☐ Wind ☐ Snow   Barometer:_____   Temp:____

I have felt: ☐ Cold   ☐ Hot   ☐ Comfortable   ☐ Mixed-bag   ☐ _____

TODAY'S FOOD & DRINK

Time	Food	How I Felt After Eating

Cravings: ☐ Sweet   ☐ Salty   ☐ Spicy   ☐ Bitter   ☐ _____

Water Consumed: OZS. (YOUR WEIGHT DIVIDED BY 2, EQUALS [GOAL] OUNCES TO DRINK DAILY.*)

Other Liquids Consumed & How I Felt

*HIGH ELEVATION & CHRONIC-PAIN PATIENTS, CALCULATE 1 QUART WATER PER 50 POUNDS OF WEIGHT.

BATHROOM EXPERIENCES

Bowels ☐ Constipation ☐ Diarrhea	☐ Formed ☐ Pain _____ Times	☐ Loose ☐ Pain _____ Times	☐ Cowpie ☐ Pain _____ Times	☐ Soup ☐ Pain _____ Times	☐ Odor? ☐ Painful Gas _____ Times
Urine ☐ Too Often ☐ Infrequent	☐ Clear ☐ Pain _____ Times	☐ Cloudy ☐ Pain _____ Times	☐ Light Yellow ☐ Pain _____ Times	☐ Dark Yellow ☐ Pain _____ Times	☐ Odor? ☐ Pain _____ Times

BASAL* TEMPERATURE / BLOOD-SUGAR NUMBERS / NOTES / ETC.

*The temperature that registers on an oral thermometer when it is placed under the armpit first thing in the morning before any activity.

NOTE: Your regular body temperature (TEMP) is written in the oval on the top of the left-hand side.

SUMMARY & THOUGHTS

SUMMARY & THOUGHTS

BLOOD PRESSURE

Date Range: _____ to _____ .

Date	Reading	Hour/Minute	Date	Reading	Hour/Minute

OXIMETER

Date Range: _____ to _____ .

Date	Oxygen	Pulse	Hour/Minute	Date	Oxygen	Pulse	Hour/Minute

TODAY'S SLEEP

(TEMP)

Last night, I went to bed at _____

I fell asleep at _____ ☐ Dreams?

I slept ☐ Well ☐ Restless ☐ Insomnia

I got up _____ times to _____

Today, I woke up at _____

I felt ☐ Rested & ready for the day

☐ Stiff ☐ Tired ☐ Sick ☐ Sore ☐ Pain

Describe _____

TODAY'S PRESCRIPTIONS AND/OR SUPPLEMENTS*

Time	Prescription/Supplement	Time	Prescription/Supplement

*WHAT YOU APPLY TO YOUR SKIN MATTERS TOO!

TODAY'S EXERCISE

Type	Time	Distance, Pounds, Repetitions, etc.
Walking		
Running		
Cycling		
Stretching		

TODAY'S ACCOMPLISHMENTS (NO MATTER HOW INSIGNIFICANT THEY MAY SEEM)

_____

_____

_____

| WEIGHT | **TODAY'S RECORD** | DATE |

Weather: ☐ Sun ☐ Clouds ☐ Rain ☐ Wind ☐ Snow   Barometer:_____   Temp:_____

I have felt: ☐ Cold   ☐ Hot   ☐ Comfortable   ☐ Mixed-bag   ☐ _____

TODAY'S FOOD & DRINK

Time	Food	How I Felt After Eating

Cravings: ☐ Sweet   ☐ Salty   ☐ Spicy   ☐ Bitter   ☐ _____

Water Consumed: ozs. (YOUR WEIGHT DIVIDED BY 2, EQUALS [GOAL] OUNCES TO DRINK DAILY.*)

Other Liquids Consumed & How I Felt

*HIGH ELEVATION & CHRONIC-PAIN PATIENTS, CALCULATE 1 QUART WATER PER 50 POUNDS OF WEIGHT.

BATHROOM EXPERIENCES

Bowels ☐ Constipation ☐ Diarrhea	☐ Formed ☐ Pain _____ Times	☐ Loose ☐ Pain _____ Times	☐ Cowpie ☐ Pain _____ Times	☐ Soup ☐ Pain _____ Times	☐ Odor? ☐ Painful Gas _____ Times
Urine ☐ Too Often ☐ Infrequent	☐ Clear ☐ Pain _____ Times	☐ Cloudy ☐ Pain _____ Times	☐ Light Yellow ☐ Pain _____ Times	☐ Dark Yellow ☐ Pain _____ Times	☐ Odor? ☐ Pain _____ Times

BASAL* TEMPERATURE / BLOOD-SUGAR NUMBERS / NOTES / ETC.

*The temperature that registers on an oral thermometer when it is placed under the armpit first thing in the morning before any activity.

NOTE: Your regular body temperature (TEMP) is written in the oval on the top of the left-hand side.

TEMP	**TODAY'S SLEEP**
Last night, I went to bed at _____	Today, I woke up at _____
I fell asleep at _____ ☐ Dreams?	I felt ☐ Rested & ready for the day
I slept ☐ Well ☐ Restless ☐ Insomnia	☐ Stiff ☐ Tired ☐ Sick ☐ Sore ☐ Pain
I got up _____ times to _____	Describe _____

TODAY'S PRESCRIPTIONS AND/OR SUPPLEMENTS*

Time	Prescription/Supplement	Time	Prescription/Supplement

*WHAT YOU APPLY TO YOUR SKIN MATTERS TOO!

TODAY'S EXERCISE

Type	Time	Distance, Pounds, Repetitions, etc.
Walking		
Running		
Cycling		
Stretching		

TODAY'S ACCOMPLISHMENTS (NO MATTER HOW INSIGNIFICANT THEY MAY SEEM)

_____

_____

_____

| WEIGHT | TODAY'S RECORD | DATE |

Weather: ☐ Sun ☐ Clouds ☐ Rain ☐ Wind ☐ Snow   Barometer:_____   Temp:_____

I have felt: ☐ Cold   ☐ Hot   ☐ Comfortable   ☐ Mixed-bag   ☐ _____

TODAY'S FOOD & DRINK

Time	Food	How I Felt After Eating

Cravings: ☐ Sweet   ☐ Salty   ☐ Spicy   ☐ Bitter   ☐ _____

Water Consumed: ozs. (YOUR WEIGHT DIVIDED BY 2, EQUALS [GOAL] OUNCES TO DRINK DAILY.*)

Other Liquids Consumed & How I Felt

*HIGH ELEVATION & CHRONIC-PAIN PATIENTS, CALCULATE 1 QUART WATER PER 50 POUNDS OF WEIGHT.

BATHROOM EXPERIENCES

Bowels ☐ Constipation ☐ Diarrhea	☐ Formed ☐ Pain _____ Times	☐ Loose ☐ Pain _____ Times	☐ Cowpie ☐ Pain _____ Times	☐ Soup ☐ Pain _____ Times	☐ Odor? ☐ Painful Gas _____ Times
Urine ☐ Too Often ☐ Infrequent	☐ Clear ☐ Pain _____ Times	☐ Cloudy ☐ Pain _____ Times	☐ Light Yellow ☐ Pain _____ Times	☐ Dark Yellow ☐ Pain _____ Times	☐ Odor? ☐ Pain _____ Times

BASAL* TEMPERATURE / BLOOD-SUGAR NUMBERS / NOTES / ETC.

*The temperature that registers on an oral thermometer when it is placed under the armpit first thing in the morning before any activity.

NOTE: Your regular body temperature (TEMP) is written in the oval on the top of the left-hand side.

TODAY'S SLEEP

TEMP

Last night, I went to bed at _____

I fell asleep at _____ ☐ Dreams?

I slept ☐ Well ☐ Restless ☐ Insomnia

I got up _____ times to _____

Today, I woke up at _____

I felt ☐ Rested & ready for the day

☐ Stiff ☐ Tired ☐ Sick ☐ Sore ☐ Pain

Describe _____

TODAY'S PRESCRIPTIONS AND/OR SUPPLEMENTS*

Time	Prescription/Supplement	Time	Prescription/Supplement

*WHAT YOU APPLY TO YOUR SKIN MATTERS TOO!

TODAY'S EXERCISE

Type	Time	Distance, Pounds, Repetitions, etc.
Walking		
Running		
Cycling		
Stretching		

TODAY'S ACCOMPLISHMENTS (NO MATTER HOW INSIGNIFICANT THEY MAY SEEM)

_____

_____

_____

| WEIGHT | **TODAY'S RECORD** | DATE |

Weather: ☐ Sun ☐ Clouds ☐ Rain ☐ Wind ☐ Snow   Barometer:_____   Temp:____

I have felt: ☐ Cold   ☐ Hot   ☐ Comfortable   ☐ Mixed-bag   ☐ _____

TODAY'S FOOD & DRINK

Time	Food	How I Felt After Eating

Cravings: ☐ Sweet   ☐ Salty   ☐ Spicy   ☐ Bitter   ☐ _____

Water Consumed: ____ ozs. (YOUR WEIGHT DIVIDED BY 2, EQUALS [GOAL] OUNCES TO DRINK DAILY.*)

Other Liquids Consumed & How I Felt

*HIGH ELEVATION & CHRONIC-PAIN PATIENTS, CALCULATE 1 QUART WATER PER 50 POUNDS OF WEIGHT.

BATHROOM EXPERIENCES

Bowels ☐ Constipation ☐ Diarrhea	☐ Formed ☐ Pain ____ Times	☐ Loose ☐ Pain ____ Times	☐ Cowpie ☐ Pain ____ Times	☐ Soup ☐ Pain ____ Times	☐ Odor? ☐ Painful Gas ____ Times
Urine ☐ Too Often ☐ Infrequent	☐ Clear ☐ Pain ____ Times	☐ Cloudy ☐ Pain ____ Times	☐ Light Yellow ☐ Pain ____ Times	☐ Dark Yellow ☐ Pain ____ Times	☐ Odor? ☐ Pain ____ Times

BASAL* TEMPERATURE / BLOOD-SUGAR NUMBERS / NOTES / ETC.

*The temperature that registers on an oral thermometer when it is placed under the armpit first thing in the morning before any activity.

NOTE: Your regular body temperature (TEMP) is written in the oval on the top of the left-hand side.

TEMP

TODAY'S SLEEP

Last night, I went to bed at _____

I fell asleep at _____ ☐ Dreams?

I slept ☐ Well ☐ Restless ☐ Insomnia

I got up _____ times to _____

Today, I woke up at _____

I felt ☐ Rested & ready for the day

☐ Stiff ☐ Tired ☐ Sick ☐ Sore ☐ Pain

Describe _____

TODAY'S PRESCRIPTIONS AND/OR SUPPLEMENTS*

Time	Prescription/Supplement	Time	Prescription/Supplement

*WHAT YOU APPLY TO YOUR SKIN MATTERS TOO!

TODAY'S EXERCISE

Type	Time	Distance, Pounds, Repetitions, etc.
Walking		
Running		
Cycling		
Stretching		

TODAY'S ACCOMPLISHMENTS (NO MATTER HOW INSIGNIFICANT THEY MAY SEEM)

_____

_____

_____

| WEIGHT | TODAY'S RECORD | DATE |

Weather: ☐ Sun ☐ Clouds ☐ Rain ☐ Wind ☐ Snow   Barometer:_____   Temp:___H__/__L__

I have felt: ☐ Cold   ☐ Hot   ☐ Comfortable   ☐ Mixed-bag   ☐ _____

TODAY'S FOOD & DRINK

Time	Food	How I Felt After Eating

Cravings: ☐ Sweet   ☐ Salty   ☐ Spicy   ☐ Bitter   ☐ _____

Water Consumed: OZS. (YOUR WEIGHT DIVIDED BY 2, EQUALS [GOAL] OUNCES TO DRINK DAILY.*)

Other Liquids Consumed & How I Felt

*HIGH ELEVATION & CHRONIC-PAIN PATIENTS, CALCULATE 1 QUART WATER PER 50 POUNDS OF WEIGHT.

BATHROOM EXPERIENCES

Bowels ☐ Constipation ☐ Diarrhea	☐ Formed ☐ Pain _____ Times	☐ Loose ☐ Pain _____ Times	☐ Cowpie ☐ Pain _____ Times	☐ Soup ☐ Pain _____ Times	☐ Odor? ☐ Painful Gas _____ Times
Urine ☐ Too Often ☐ Infrequent	☐ Clear ☐ Pain _____ Times	☐ Cloudy ☐ Pain _____ Times	☐ Light Yellow ☐ Pain _____ Times	☐ Dark Yellow ☐ Pain _____ Times	☐ Odor? ☐ Pain _____ Times

BASAL* TEMPERATURE / BLOOD-SUGAR NUMBERS / NOTES / ETC.

*The temperature that registers on an oral thermometer when it is placed under the armpit first thing in the morning before any activity.

NOTE: Your regular body temperature (TEMP) is written in the oval on the top of the left-hand side.

(TEMP) **TODAY'S SLEEP**

Last night, I went to bed at _____ Today, I woke up at _____

I fell asleep at _____ ☐ Dreams? I felt ☐ Rested & ready for the day

I slept ☐ Well ☐ Restless ☐ Insomnia ☐ Stiff ☐ Tired ☐ Sick ☐ Sore ☐ Pain

I got up _____ times to _____ Describe _____

TODAY'S PRESCRIPTIONS AND/OR SUPPLEMENTS*

Time	Prescription/Supplement	Time	Prescription/Supplement

*WHAT YOU APPLY TO YOUR SKIN MATTERS TOO!

TODAY'S EXERCISE

Type	Time	Distance, Pounds, Repetitions, etc.
Walking		
Running		
Cycling		
Stretching		

TODAY'S ACCOMPLISHMENTS (NO MATTER HOW INSIGNIFICANT THEY MAY SEEM)

_____

_____

_____

TODAY'S RECORD

WEIGHT   **DATE**

Weather: ☐ Sun ☐ Clouds ☐ Rain ☐ Wind ☐ Snow   Barometer:_____   Temp:____ / ____

I have felt: ☐ Cold   ☐ Hot   ☐ Comfortable   ☐ Mixed-bag   ☐ _____

TODAY'S FOOD & DRINK

Time	Food	How I Felt After Eating

Cravings: ☐ Sweet   ☐ Salty   ☐ Spicy   ☐ Bitter   ☐ _____

Water Consumed: ozs.   (YOUR WEIGHT DIVIDED BY 2, EQUALS [GOAL] OUNCES TO DRINK DAILY.*)

Other Liquids Consumed & How I Felt

*HIGH ELEVATION & CHRONIC-PAIN PATIENTS, CALCULATE 1 QUART WATER PER 50 POUNDS OF WEIGHT.

BATHROOM EXPERIENCES

Bowels ☐ Constipation ☐ Diarrhea	☐ Formed ☐ Pain _____ Times	☐ Loose ☐ Pain _____ Times	☐ Cowpie ☐ Pain _____ Times	☐ Soup ☐ Pain _____ Times	☐ Odor? ☐ Painful Gas _____ Times
Urine ☐ Too Often ☐ Infrequent	☐ Clear ☐ Pain _____ Times	☐ Cloudy ☐ Pain _____ Times	☐ Light Yellow ☐ Pain _____ Times	☐ Dark Yellow ☐ Pain _____ Times	☐ Odor? ☐ Pain _____ Times

BASAL* TEMPERATURE / BLOOD-SUGAR NUMBERS / NOTES / ETC.

*The temperature that registers on an oral thermometer when it is placed under the armpit first thing in the morning before any activity.

NOTE: Your regular body temperature (TEMP) is written in the oval on the top of the left-hand side.

TEMP

TODAY'S SLEEP

Last night, I went to bed at _____

I fell asleep at _____ ☐ Dreams?

I slept ☐ Well ☐ Restless ☐ Insomnia

I got up _____ times to _____

Today, I woke up at _____

I felt ☐ Rested & ready for the day

☐ Stiff ☐ Tired ☐ Sick ☐ Sore ☐ Pain

Describe _____

TODAY'S PRESCRIPTIONS AND/OR SUPPLEMENTS*

Time	Prescription/Supplement	Time	Prescription/Supplement

*WHAT YOU APPLY TO YOUR SKIN MATTERS TOO!

TODAY'S EXERCISE

Type	Time	Distance, Pounds, Repetitions, etc.
Walking		
Running		
Cycling		
Stretching		

TODAY'S ACCOMPLISHMENTS (NO MATTER HOW INSIGNIFICANT THEY MAY SEEM)

_____

_____

_____

WEIGHT | TODAY'S RECORD | DATE

Weather: ☐ Sun ☐ Clouds ☐ Rain ☐ Wind ☐ Snow   Barometer:_____   Temp:_____

I have felt: ☐ Cold   ☐ Hot   ☐ Comfortable   ☐ Mixed-bag   ☐ _____

TODAY'S FOOD & DRINK

Time	Food	How I Felt After Eating

Cravings: ☐ Sweet   ☐ Salty   ☐ Spicy   ☐ Bitter   ☐ _____

Water Consumed: OZS.   (YOUR WEIGHT DIVIDED BY 2, EQUALS [GOAL] OUNCES TO DRINK DAILY.*)

Other Liquids Consumed & How I Felt

*HIGH ELEVATION & CHRONIC-PAIN PATIENTS, CALCULATE 1 QUART WATER PER 50 POUNDS OF WEIGHT.

BATHROOM EXPERIENCES

Bowels ☐ Constipation ☐ Diarrhea	☐ Formed ☐ Pain _____ Times	☐ Loose ☐ Pain _____ Times	☐ Cowpie ☐ Pain _____ Times	☐ Soup ☐ Pain _____ Times	☐ Odor? ☐ Painful Gas _____ Times
Urine ☐ Too Often ☐ Infrequent	☐ Clear ☐ Pain _____ Times	☐ Cloudy ☐ Pain _____ Times	☐ Light Yellow ☐ Pain _____ Times	☐ Dark Yellow ☐ Pain _____ Times	☐ Odor? ☐ Pain _____ Times

BASAL* TEMPERATURE / BLOOD-SUGAR NUMBERS / NOTES / ETC.

*The temperature that registers on an oral thermometer when it is placed under the armpit first thing in the morning before any activity.

NOTE: Your regular body temperature (TEMP) is written in the oval on the top of the left-hand side.

TODAY'S SLEEP

(TEMP)

Last night, I went to bed at _____

I fell asleep at _____ ☐ Dreams?

I slept ☐ Well ☐ Restless ☐ Insomnia

I got up _____ times to _____

Today, I woke up at _____

I felt ☐ Rested & ready for the day

☐ Stiff ☐ Tired ☐ Sick ☐ Sore ☐ Pain

Describe _____

TODAY'S PRESCRIPTIONS AND/OR SUPPLEMENTS*

Time	Prescription/Supplement	Time	Prescription/Supplement

*WHAT YOU APPLY TO YOUR SKIN MATTERS TOO!

TODAY'S EXERCISE

Type	Time	Distance, Pounds, Repetitions, etc.
Walking		
Running		
Cycling		
Stretching		

TODAY'S ACCOMPLISHMENTS (NO MATTER HOW INSIGNIFICANT THEY MAY SEEM)

_____

_____

_____

TODAY'S RECORD

WEIGHT   **DATE**

Weather: ☐ Sun ☐ Clouds ☐ Rain ☐ Wind ☐ Snow Barometer:_____ Temp:____

I have felt: ☐ Cold ☐ Hot ☐ Comfortable ☐ Mixed-bag ☐ _____

TODAY'S FOOD & DRINK

Time	Food	How I Felt After Eating

Cravings: ☐ Sweet ☐ Salty ☐ Spicy ☐ Bitter ☐ _____

Water Consumed: _____ ozs. (YOUR WEIGHT DIVIDED BY 2, EQUALS [GOAL] OUNCES TO DRINK DAILY.*)

Other Liquids Consumed & How I Felt

*HIGH ELEVATION & CHRONIC-PAIN PATIENTS, CALCULATE 1 QUART WATER PER 50 POUNDS OF WEIGHT.

BATHROOM EXPERIENCES

Bowels ☐ Constipation ☐ Diarrhea	☐ Formed ☐ Pain _____ Times	☐ Loose ☐ Pain _____ Times	☐ Cowpie ☐ Pain _____ Times	☐ Soup ☐ Pain _____ Times	☐ Odor? ☐ Painful Gas _____ Times
Urine ☐ Too Often ☐ Infrequent	☐ Clear ☐ Pain _____ Times	☐ Cloudy ☐ Pain _____ Times	☐ Light Yellow ☐ Pain _____ Times	☐ Dark Yellow ☐ Pain _____ Times	☐ Odor? ☐ Pain _____ Times

BASAL* TEMPERATURE / BLOOD-SUGAR NUMBERS / NOTES / ETC.

*The temperature that registers on an oral thermometer when it is placed under the armpit first thing in the morning before any activity.

NOTE: Your regular body temperature (TEMP) is written in the oval on the top of the left-hand side.

TEMP	**TODAY'S SLEEP**

Last night, I went to bed at _____   Today, I woke up at _____

I fell asleep at _____ ☐ Dreams?   I felt ☐ Rested & ready for the day

I slept ☐ Well ☐ Restless ☐ Insomnia   ☐ Stiff ☐ Tired ☐ Sick ☐ Sore ☐ Pain

I got up _____ times to _____   Describe _____

TODAY'S PRESCRIPTIONS AND/OR SUPPLEMENTS*

Time	Prescription/Supplement	Time	Prescription/Supplement

WHAT YOU APPLY TO YOUR SKIN MATTERS TOO!

TODAY'S EXERCISE

Type	Time	Distance, Pounds, Repetitions, etc.
Walking		
Running		
Cycling		
Stretching		

TODAY'S ACCOMPLISHMENTS (NO MATTER HOW INSIGNIFICANT THEY MAY SEEM)

_____

_____

_____

| WEIGHT | TODAY'S RECORD | DATE |

Weather: ☐ Sun ☐ Clouds ☐ Rain ☐ Wind ☐ Snow   Barometer:_____   Temp: ___H_/_L_

I have felt: ☐ Cold   ☐ Hot   ☐ Comfortable   ☐ Mixed-bag   ☐ _____

TODAY'S FOOD & DRINK

Time	Food	How I Felt After Eating

Cravings: ☐ Sweet   ☐ Salty   ☐ Spicy   ☐ Bitter   ☐ _____

Water Consumed: _____ ozs. (YOUR WEIGHT DIVIDED BY 2, EQUALS [GOAL] OUNCES TO DRINK DAILY.*)

Other Liquids Consumed & How I Felt

*HIGH ELEVATION & CHRONIC-PAIN PATIENTS, CALCULATE 1 QUART WATER PER 50 POUNDS OF WEIGHT.

BATHROOM EXPERIENCES

Bowels ☐ Constipation ☐ Diarrhea	☐ Formed ☐ Pain _____ Times	☐ Loose ☐ Pain _____ Times	☐ Cowpie ☐ Pain _____ Times	☐ Soup ☐ Pain _____ Times	☐ Odor? ☐ Painful Gas _____ Times
Urine ☐ Too Often ☐ Infrequent	☐ Clear ☐ Pain _____ Times	☐ Cloudy ☐ Pain _____ Times	☐ Light Yellow ☐ Pain _____ Times	☐ Dark Yellow ☐ Pain _____ Times	☐ Odor? ☐ Pain _____ Times

BASAL* TEMPERATURE / BLOOD-SUGAR NUMBERS / NOTES / ETC.

*The temperature that registers on an oral thermometer when it is placed under the armpit first thing in the morning before any activity.

NOTE: Your regular body temperature (TEMP) is written in the oval on the top of the left-hand side.

TEMP

TODAY'S SLEEP

Last night, I went to bed at _____

I fell asleep at _____ ☐ Dreams?

I slept ☐ Well ☐ Restless ☐ Insomnia

I got up _____ times to _____

Today, I woke up at _____

I felt ☐ Rested & ready for the day

☐ Stiff ☐ Tired ☐ Sick ☐ Sore ☐ Pain

Describe _____

TODAY'S PRESCRIPTIONS AND/OR SUPPLEMENTS*

Time	Prescription/Supplement	Time	Prescription/Supplement

*WHAT YOU APPLY TO YOUR SKIN MATTERS TOO!

TODAY'S EXERCISE

Type	Time	Distance, Pounds, Repetitions, etc.
Walking		
Running		
Cycling		
Stretching		

TODAY'S ACCOMPLISHMENTS (NO MATTER HOW INSIGNIFICANT THEY MAY SEEM)

_____

_____

_____

WEIGHT	TODAY'S RECORD	DATE

Weather: ☐ Sun ☐ Clouds ☐ Rain ☐ Wind ☐ Snow Barometer:_____ Temp:_____

I have felt: ☐ Cold ☐ Hot ☐ Comfortable ☐ Mixed-bag ☐ _____

TODAY'S FOOD & DRINK

Time	Food	How I Felt After Eating

Cravings: ☐ Sweet ☐ Salty ☐ Spicy ☐ Bitter ☐ _____

Water Consumed: ____ ozs. (YOUR WEIGHT DIVIDED BY 2, EQUALS [GOAL] OUNCES TO DRINK DAILY.*)

Other Liquids Consumed & How I Felt

*HIGH ELEVATION & CHRONIC-PAIN PATIENTS, CALCULATE 1 QUART WATER PER 50 POUNDS OF WEIGHT.

BATHROOM EXPERIENCES

Bowels ☐ Constipation ☐ Diarrhea	☐ Formed ☐ Pain _____ Times	☐ Loose ☐ Pain _____ Times	☐ Cowpie ☐ Pain _____ Times	☐ Soup ☐ Pain _____ Times	☐ Odor? ☐ Painful Gas _____ Times
Urine ☐ Too Often ☐ Infrequent	☐ Clear ☐ Pain _____ Times	☐ Cloudy ☐ Pain _____ Times	☐ Light Yellow ☐ Pain _____ Times	☐ Dark Yellow ☐ Pain _____ Times	☐ Odor? ☐ Pain _____ Times

BASAL* TEMPERATURE / BLOOD-SUGAR NUMBERS / NOTES / ETC.

*The temperature that registers on an oral thermometer when it is placed under the armpit first thing in the morning before any activity.

NOTE: Your regular body temperature (TEMP) is written in the oval on the top of the left-hand side.

TEMP

TODAY'S SLEEP

Last night, I went to bed at _____

I fell asleep at _____ ☐ Dreams?

I slept ☐ Well ☐ Restless ☐ Insomnia

I got up _____ times to _____

Today, I woke up at _____

I felt ☐ Rested & ready for the day

☐ Stiff ☐ Tired ☐ Sick ☐ Sore ☐ Pain

Describe _____

TODAY'S PRESCRIPTIONS AND/OR SUPPLEMENTS*

Time	Prescription/Supplement	Time	Prescription/Supplement

*WHAT YOU APPLY TO YOUR SKIN MATTERS TOO!

TODAY'S EXERCISE

Type	Time	Distance, Pounds, Repetitions, etc.
Walking		
Running		
Cycling		
Stretching		

TODAY'S ACCOMPLISHMENTS (NO MATTER HOW INSIGNIFICANT THEY MAY SEEM)

_____

_____

_____

WEIGHT	TODAY'S RECORD	DATE

Weather: ☐ Sun ☐ Clouds ☐ Rain ☐ Wind ☐ Snow   Barometer:_____   Temp:_____

I have felt: ☐ Cold   ☐ Hot   ☐ Comfortable   ☐ Mixed-bag   ☐ _____

TODAY'S FOOD & DRINK

Time	Food	How I Felt After Eating

Cravings: ☐ Sweet   ☐ Salty   ☐ Spicy   ☐ Bitter   ☐ _____

Water Consumed: ozs. (YOUR WEIGHT DIVIDED BY 2, EQUALS [GOAL] OUNCES TO DRINK DAILY.*)

Other Liquids Consumed & How I Felt

*HIGH ELEVATION & CHRONIC-PAIN PATIENTS, CALCULATE 1 QUART WATER PER 50 POUNDS OF WEIGHT.

BATHROOM EXPERIENCES

Bowels ☐ Constipation ☐ Diarrhea	☐ Formed ☐ Pain ____ Times	☐ Loose ☐ Pain ____ Times	☐ Cowpie ☐ Pain ____ Times	☐ Soup ☐ Pain ____ Times	☐ Odor? ☐ Painful Gas ____ Times
Urine ☐ Too Often ☐ Infrequent	☐ Clear ☐ Pain ____ Times	☐ Cloudy ☐ Pain ____ Times	☐ Light Yellow ☐ Pain ____ Times	☐ Dark Yellow ☐ Pain ____ Times	☐ Odor? ☐ Pain ____ Times

BASAL* TEMPERATURE / BLOOD-SUGAR NUMBERS / NOTES / ETC.

*The temperature that registers on an oral thermometer when it is placed under the armpit first thing in the morning before any activity.

NOTE: Your regular body temperature (TEMP) is written in the oval on the top of the left-hand side.

(TEMP)

TODAY'S SLEEP

Last night, I went to bed at _____

I fell asleep at _____ ☐ Dreams?

I slept ☐ Well ☐ Restless ☐ Insomnia

I got up _____ times to _____

Today, I woke up at _____

I felt ☐ Rested & ready for the day

☐ Stiff ☐ Tired ☐ Sick ☐ Sore ☐ Pain

Describe _____

TODAY'S PRESCRIPTIONS AND/OR SUPPLEMENTS*

Time	Prescription/Supplement	Time	Prescription/Supplement

*WHAT YOU APPLY TO YOUR SKIN MATTERS TOO!

TODAY'S EXERCISE

Type	Time	Distance, Pounds, Repetitions, etc.
Walking		
Running		
Cycling		
Stretching		

TODAY'S ACCOMPLISHMENTS (NO MATTER HOW INSIGNIFICANT THEY MAY SEEM)

_____

_____

_____

WEIGHT	TODAY'S RECORD	DATE

Weather: ☐ Sun ☐ Clouds ☐ Rain ☐ Wind ☐ Snow   Barometer: _____   Temp: _____

I have felt: ☐ Cold   ☐ Hot   ☐ Comfortable   ☐ Mixed-bag   ☐ _____

TODAY'S FOOD & DRINK

Time	Food	How I Felt After Eating

Cravings: ☐ Sweet   ☐ Salty   ☐ Spicy   ☐ Bitter   ☐ _____

Water Consumed: ozs.   (YOUR WEIGHT DIVIDED BY 2, EQUALS [GOAL] OUNCES TO DRINK DAILY.*)

Other Liquids Consumed & How I Felt

*HIGH ELEVATION & CHRONIC-PAIN PATIENTS, CALCULATE 1 QUART WATER PER 50 POUNDS OF WEIGHT.

BATHROOM EXPERIENCES

Bowels ☐ Constipation ☐ Diarrhea	☐ Formed ☐ Pain _____ Times	☐ Loose ☐ Pain _____ Times	☐ Cowpie ☐ Pain _____ Times	☐ Soup ☐ Pain _____ Times	☐ Odor? ☐ Painful Gas _____ Times
Urine ☐ Too Often ☐ Infrequent	☐ Clear ☐ Pain _____ Times	☐ Cloudy ☐ Pain _____ Times	☐ Light Yellow ☐ Pain _____ Times	☐ Dark Yellow ☐ Pain _____ Times	☐ Odor? ☐ Pain _____ Times

BASAL* TEMPERATURE / BLOOD-SUGAR NUMBERS / NOTES / ETC.

*The temperature that registers on an oral thermometer when it is placed under the armpit first thing in the morning before any activity.

NOTE: Your regular body temperature (TEMP) is written in the oval on the top of the left-hand side.

TODAY'S SLEEP

(TEMP)

Last night, I went to bed at _____

I fell asleep at _____ ☐ Dreams?

I slept ☐ Well ☐ Restless ☐ Insomnia

I got up _____ times to _____

Today, I woke up at _____

I felt ☐ Rested & ready for the day

☐ Stiff ☐ Tired ☐ Sick ☐ Sore ☐ Pain

Describe _____

TODAY'S PRESCRIPTIONS AND/OR SUPPLEMENTS*

Time	Prescription/Supplement	Time	Prescription/Supplement

*WHAT YOU APPLY TO YOUR SKIN MATTERS TOO!

TODAY'S EXERCISE

Type	Time	Distance, Pounds, Repetitions, etc.
Walking		
Running		
Cycling		
Stretching		

TODAY'S ACCOMPLISHMENTS (NO MATTER HOW INSIGNIFICANT THEY MAY SEEM)

_____

_____

_____

(WEIGHT) TODAY'S RECORD (DATE)

Weather: ☐ Sun ☐ Clouds ☐ Rain ☐ Wind ☐ Snow Barometer:_____ Temp:____H____L

I have felt: ☐ Cold ☐ Hot ☐ Comfortable ☐ Mixed-bag ☐ _____

TODAY'S FOOD & DRINK

Time	Food	How I Felt After Eating

Cravings: ☐ Sweet ☐ Salty ☐ Spicy ☐ Bitter ☐ _____

Water Consumed: OZS. (YOUR WEIGHT DIVIDED BY 2, EQUALS [GOAL] OUNCES TO DRINK DAILY.*)

Other Liquids Consumed & How I Felt

*HIGH ELEVATION & CHRONIC-PAIN PATIENTS, CALCULATE 1 QUART WATER PER 50 POUNDS OF WEIGHT.

BATHROOM EXPERIENCES

Bowels ☐ Constipation ☐ Diarrhea	☐ Formed ☐ Pain _____ Times	☐ Loose ☐ Pain _____ Times	☐ Cowpie ☐ Pain _____ Times	☐ Soup ☐ Pain _____ Times	☐ Odor? ☐ Painful Gas _____ Times
Urine ☐ Too Often ☐ Infrequent	☐ Clear ☐ Pain _____ Times	☐ Cloudy ☐ Pain _____ Times	☐ Light Yellow ☐ Pain _____ Times	☐ Dark Yellow ☐ Pain _____ Times	☐ Odor? ☐ Pain _____ Times

BASAL* TEMPERATURE / BLOOD-SUGAR NUMBERS / NOTES / ETC.

*The temperature that registers on an oral thermometer when it is placed under the armpit first thing in the morning before any activity.

NOTE: Your regular body temperature (TEMP) is written in the oval on the top of the left-hand side.

TEMP | TODAY'S SLEEP

Last night, I went to bed at _____

I fell asleep at _____ ☐ Dreams?

I slept ☐ Well ☐ Restless ☐ Insomnia

I got up _____ times to _____

Today, I woke up at _____

I felt ☐ Rested & ready for the day

☐ Stiff ☐ Tired ☐ Sick ☐ Sore ☐ Pain

Describe _____

TODAY'S PRESCRIPTIONS AND/OR SUPPLEMENTS*

Time	Prescription/Supplement	Time	Prescription/Supplement

*WHAT YOU APPLY TO YOUR SKIN MATTERS TOO!

TODAY'S EXERCISE

Type	Time	Distance, Pounds, Repetitions, etc.
Walking		
Running		
Cycling		
Stretching		

TODAY'S ACCOMPLISHMENTS (NO MATTER HOW INSIGNIFICANT THEY MAY SEEM)

_____

_____

_____

WEIGHT	TODAY'S RECORD	DATE

Weather: ☐ Sun ☐ Clouds ☐ Rain ☐ Wind ☐ Snow   Barometer:_____   Temp:_____

I have felt: ☐ Cold   ☐ Hot   ☐ Comfortable   ☐ Mixed-bag   ☐ _____

TODAY'S FOOD & DRINK

Time	Food	How I Felt After Eating

Cravings: ☐ Sweet   ☐ Salty   ☐ Spicy   ☐ Bitter   ☐ _____

Water Consumed: _____ OZS. (YOUR WEIGHT DIVIDED BY 2, EQUALS [GOAL] OUNCES TO DRINK DAILY.*)

Other Liquids Consumed & How I Felt

*HIGH ELEVATION & CHRONIC-PAIN PATIENTS, CALCULATE 1 QUART WATER PER 50 POUNDS OF WEIGHT.

BATHROOM EXPERIENCES

Bowels ☐ Constipation ☐ Diarrhea	☐ Formed ☐ Pain _____ Times	☐ Loose ☐ Pain _____ Times	☐ Cowpie ☐ Pain _____ Times	☐ Soup ☐ Pain _____ Times	☐ Odor? ☐ Painful Gas _____ Times
Urine ☐ Too Often ☐ Infrequent	☐ Clear ☐ Pain _____ Times	☐ Cloudy ☐ Pain _____ Times	☐ Light Yellow ☐ Pain _____ Times	☐ Dark Yellow ☐ Pain _____ Times	☐ Odor? ☐ Pain _____ Times

BASAL* TEMPERATURE / BLOOD-SUGAR NUMBERS / NOTES / ETC.

*The temperature that registers on an oral thermometer when it is placed under the armpit first thing in the morning before any activity.

NOTE: Your regular body temperature (TEMP) is written in the oval on the top of the left-hand side.

(TEMP)

TODAY'S SLEEP

Last night, I went to bed at _____

I fell asleep at _____ ☐ Dreams?

I slept ☐ Well ☐ Restless ☐ Insomnia

I got up _____ times to _____

Today, I woke up at _____

I felt ☐ Rested & ready for the day

☐ Stiff ☐ Tired ☐ Sick ☐ Sore ☐ Pain

Describe _____

TODAY'S PRESCRIPTIONS AND/OR SUPPLEMENTS*

Time	Prescription/Supplement	Time	Prescription/Supplement

*WHAT YOU APPLY TO YOUR SKIN MATTERS TOO!

TODAY'S EXERCISE

Type	Time	Distance, Pounds, Repetitions, etc.
Walking		
Running		
Cycling		
Stretching		

TODAY'S ACCOMPLISHMENTS (NO MATTER HOW INSIGNIFICANT THEY MAY SEEM)

_____

_____

_____

| WEIGHT | TODAY'S RECORD | DATE |

Weather: ☐ Sun ☐ Clouds ☐ Rain ☐ Wind ☐ Snow   Barometer:_____   Temp:____ / ____

I have felt: ☐ Cold ☐ Hot ☐ Comfortable ☐ Mixed-bag ☐ _____

TODAY'S FOOD & DRINK

Time	Food	How I Felt After Eating

Cravings: ☐ Sweet ☐ Salty ☐ Spicy ☐ Bitter ☐ _____

Water Consumed: _____ ozs. (YOUR WEIGHT DIVIDED BY 2, EQUALS [GOAL] OUNCES TO DRINK DAILY.*)

Other Liquids Consumed & How I Felt

*HIGH ELEVATION & CHRONIC-PAIN PATIENTS, CALCULATE 1 QUART WATER PER 50 POUNDS OF WEIGHT.

BATHROOM EXPERIENCES

Bowels ☐ Constipation ☐ Diarrhea	☐ Formed ☐ Pain _____ Times	☐ Loose ☐ Pain _____ Times	☐ Cowpie ☐ Pain _____ Times	☐ Soup ☐ Pain _____ Times	☐ Odor? ☐ Painful Gas _____ Times
Urine ☐ Too Often ☐ Infrequent	☐ Clear ☐ Pain _____ Times	☐ Cloudy ☐ Pain _____ Times	☐ Light Yellow ☐ Pain _____ Times	☐ Dark Yellow ☐ Pain _____ Times	☐ Odor? ☐ Pain _____ Times

BASAL* TEMPERATURE / BLOOD-SUGAR NUMBERS / NOTES / ETC.

*The temperature that registers on an oral thermometer when it is placed under the armpit first thing in the morning before any activity.

NOTE: Your regular body temperature (TEMP) is written in the oval on the top of the left-hand side.

(TEMP)

TODAY'S SLEEP

Last night, I went to bed at _____

I fell asleep at _____ ☐ Dreams?

I slept ☐ Well ☐ Restless ☐ Insomnia

I got up _____ times to _____

Today, I woke up at _____

I felt ☐ Rested & ready for the day

☐ Stiff ☐ Tired ☐ Sick ☐ Sore ☐ Pain

Describe _____

TODAY'S PRESCRIPTIONS AND/OR SUPPLEMENTS*

Time	Prescription/Supplement	Time	Prescription/Supplement

*WHAT YOU APPLY TO YOUR SKIN MATTERS TOO!

TODAY'S EXERCISE

Type	Time	Distance, Pounds, Repetitions, etc.
Walking		
Running		
Cycling		
Stretching		

TODAY'S ACCOMPLISHMENTS (NO MATTER HOW INSIGNIFICANT THEY MAY SEEM)

_____

_____

_____

| WEIGHT | TODAY'S RECORD | DATE |

Weather: ☐ Sun ☐ Clouds ☐ Rain ☐ Wind ☐ Snow Barometer:_____ Temp:____

I have felt: ☐ Cold ☐ Hot ☐ Comfortable ☐ Mixed-bag ☐ _____

TODAY'S FOOD & DRINK

Time	Food	How I Felt After Eating

Cravings: ☐ Sweet ☐ Salty ☐ Spicy ☐ Bitter ☐ _____

Water Consumed: _____ ozs. (YOUR WEIGHT DIVIDED BY 2, EQUALS [GOAL] OUNCES TO DRINK DAILY.*)

Other Liquids Consumed & How I Felt

*HIGH ELEVATION & CHRONIC-PAIN PATIENTS, CALCULATE 1 QUART WATER PER 50 POUNDS OF WEIGHT.

BATHROOM EXPERIENCES

Bowels ☐ Constipation ☐ Diarrhea	☐ Formed ☐ Pain _____ Times	☐ Loose ☐ Pain _____ Times	☐ Cowpie ☐ Pain _____ Times	☐ Soup ☐ Pain _____ Times	☐ Odor? ☐ Painful Gas _____ Times
Urine ☐ Too Often ☐ Infrequent	☐ Clear ☐ Pain _____ Times	☐ Cloudy ☐ Pain _____ Times	☐ Light Yellow ☐ Pain _____ Times	☐ Dark Yellow ☐ Pain _____ Times	☐ Odor? ☐ Pain _____ Times

BASAL* TEMPERATURE / BLOOD-SUGAR NUMBERS / NOTES / ETC.

*The temperature that registers on an oral thermometer when it is placed under the armpit first thing in the morning before any activity.

NOTE: Your regular body temperature (TEMP) is written in the oval on the top of the left-hand side.

TEMP

TODAY'S SLEEP

Last night, I went to bed at _____

I fell asleep at _____ ☐ Dreams?

I slept ☐ Well ☐ Restless ☐ Insomnia

I got up _____ times to _____

Today, I woke up at _____

I felt ☐ Rested & ready for the day

☐ Stiff ☐ Tired ☐ Sick ☐ Sore ☐ Pain

Describe _____

TODAY'S PRESCRIPTIONS AND/OR SUPPLEMENTS*

Time	Prescription/Supplement	Time	Prescription/Supplement

*WHAT YOU APPLY TO YOUR SKIN MATTERS TOO!

TODAY'S EXERCISE

Type	Time	Distance, Pounds, Repetitions, etc.
Walking		
Running		
Cycling		
Stretching		

TODAY'S ACCOMPLISHMENTS (NO MATTER HOW INSIGNIFICANT THEY MAY SEEM)

_____

_____

_____

| WEIGHT | TODAY'S RECORD | DATE |

Weather: ☐ Sun ☐ Clouds ☐ Rain ☐ Wind ☐ Snow   Barometer:_____   Temp:_____

I have felt: ☐ Cold   ☐ Hot   ☐ Comfortable   ☐ Mixed-bag   ☐ _____

TODAY'S FOOD & DRINK

Time	Food	How I Felt After Eating

Cravings: ☐ Sweet   ☐ Salty   ☐ Spicy   ☐ Bitter   ☐ _____

Water Consumed: ozs. (YOUR WEIGHT DIVIDED BY 2, EQUALS [GOAL] OUNCES TO DRINK DAILY.*)

Other Liquids Consumed & How I Felt

*HIGH ELEVATION & CHRONIC-PAIN PATIENTS, CALCULATE 1 QUART WATER PER 50 POUNDS OF WEIGHT.

BATHROOM EXPERIENCES

Bowels ☐ Constipation ☐ Diarrhea	☐ Formed ☐ Pain _____ Times	☐ Loose ☐ Pain _____ Times	☐ Cowpie ☐ Pain _____ Times	☐ Soup ☐ Pain _____ Times	☐ Odor? ☐ Painful Gas _____ Times
Urine ☐ Too Often ☐ Infrequent	☐ Clear ☐ Pain _____ Times	☐ Cloudy ☐ Pain _____ Times	☐ Light Yellow ☐ Pain _____ Times	☐ Dark Yellow ☐ Pain _____ Times	☐ Odor? ☐ Pain _____ Times

BASAL* TEMPERATURE / BLOOD-SUGAR NUMBERS / NOTES / ETC.

*The temperature that registers on an oral thermometer when it is placed under the armpit first thing in the morning before any activity.

NOTE: Your regular body temperature (TEMP) is written in the oval on the top of the left-hand side.

(TEMP)

TODAY'S SLEEP

Last night, I went to bed at _____

I fell asleep at _____ ☐ Dreams?

I slept ☐ Well ☐ Restless ☐ Insomnia

I got up _____ times to _____

Today, I woke up at _____

I felt ☐ Rested & ready for the day

☐ Stiff ☐ Tired ☐ Sick ☐ Sore ☐ Pain

Describe _____

TODAY'S PRESCRIPTIONS AND/OR SUPPLEMENTS*

Time	Prescription/Supplement	Time	Prescription/Supplement

*WHAT YOU APPLY TO YOUR SKIN MATTERS TOO!

TODAY'S EXERCISE

Type	Time	Distance, Pounds, Repetitions, etc.
Walking		
Running		
Cycling		
Stretching		

TODAY'S ACCOMPLISHMENTS (NO MATTER HOW INSIGNIFICANT THEY MAY SEEM)

_____

_____

_____

| WEIGHT | TODAY'S RECORD | DATE |

Weather: ☐ Sun ☐ Clouds ☐ Rain ☐ Wind ☐ Snow   Barometer:_____   Temp:_____

I have felt: ☐ Cold   ☐ Hot   ☐ Comfortable   ☐ Mixed-bag   ☐ _____

TODAY'S FOOD & DRINK

Time	Food	How I Felt After Eating

Cravings: ☐ Sweet   ☐ Salty   ☐ Spicy   ☐ Bitter   ☐ _____

Water Consumed: _____ ozs. (YOUR WEIGHT DIVIDED BY 2, EQUALS [GOAL] OUNCES TO DRINK DAILY.*)

Other Liquids Consumed & How I Felt

*HIGH ELEVATION & CHRONIC-PAIN PATIENTS, CALCULATE 1 QUART WATER PER 50 POUNDS OF WEIGHT.

BATHROOM EXPERIENCES

Bowels ☐ Constipation ☐ Diarrhea	☐ Formed ☐ Pain _____ Times	☐ Loose ☐ Pain _____ Times	☐ Cowpie ☐ Pain _____ Times	☐ Soup ☐ Pain _____ Times	☐ Odor? ☐ Painful Gas _____ Times
Urine ☐ Too Often ☐ Infrequent	☐ Clear ☐ Pain _____ Times	☐ Cloudy ☐ Pain _____ Times	☐ Light Yellow ☐ Pain _____ Times	☐ Dark Yellow ☐ Pain _____ Times	☐ Odor? ☐ Pain _____ Times

BASAL* TEMPERATURE / BLOOD-SUGAR NUMBERS / NOTES / ETC.

*The temperature that registers on an oral thermometer when it is placed under the armpit first thing in the morning before any activity.

NOTE: Your regular body temperature (TEMP) is written in the oval on the top of the left-hand side.

(TEMP)

TODAY'S SLEEP

Last night, I went to bed at _____

I fell asleep at _____ ☐ Dreams?

I slept ☐ Well ☐ Restless ☐ Insomnia

I got up _____ times to _____

Today, I woke up at _____

I felt ☐ Rested & ready for the day

☐ Stiff ☐ Tired ☐ Sick ☐ Sore ☐ Pain

Describe _____

TODAY'S PRESCRIPTIONS AND/OR SUPPLEMENTS*

Time	Prescription/Supplement	Time	Prescription/Supplement

*WHAT YOU APPLY TO YOUR SKIN MATTERS TOO!

TODAY'S EXERCISE

Type	Time	Distance, Pounds, Repetitions, etc.
Walking		
Running		
Cycling		
Stretching		

TODAY'S ACCOMPLISHMENTS (NO MATTER HOW INSIGNIFICANT THEY MAY SEEM)

_____

_____

_____

WEIGHT	TODAY'S RECORD	DATE

Weather: ☐ Sun ☐ Clouds ☐ Rain ☐ Wind ☐ Snow   Barometer:_____   Temp:___H__/__L__

I have felt: ☐ Cold   ☐ Hot   ☐ Comfortable   ☐ Mixed-bag   ☐ _____

TODAY'S FOOD & DRINK

Time	Food	How I Felt After Eating

Cravings: ☐ Sweet   ☐ Salty   ☐ Spicy   ☐ Bitter   ☐ _____

Water Consumed: ozs. (YOUR WEIGHT DIVIDED BY 2, EQUALS [GOAL] OUNCES TO DRINK DAILY.*)

Other Liquids Consumed & How I Felt

*HIGH ELEVATION & CHRONIC-PAIN PATIENTS, CALCULATE 1 QUART WATER PER 50 POUNDS OF WEIGHT.

BATHROOM EXPERIENCES

Bowels ☐ Constipation ☐ Diarrhea	☐ Formed ☐ Pain _____ Times	☐ Loose ☐ Pain _____ Times	☐ Cowpie ☐ Pain _____ Times	☐ Soup ☐ Pain _____ Times	☐ Odor? ☐ Painful Gas _____ Times
Urine ☐ Too Often ☐ Infrequent	☐ Clear ☐ Pain _____ Times	☐ Cloudy ☐ Pain _____ Times	☐ Light Yellow ☐ Pain _____ Times	☐ Dark Yellow ☐ Pain _____ Times	☐ Odor? ☐ Pain _____ Times

BASAL* TEMPERATURE / BLOOD-SUGAR NUMBERS / NOTES / ETC.

*The temperature that registers on an oral thermometer when it is placed under the armpit first thing in the morning before any activity.

NOTE: Your regular body temperature (TEMP) is written in the oval on the top of the left-hand side.

(TEMP)

TODAY'S SLEEP

Last night, I went to bed at _____ Today, I woke up at _____

I fell asleep at _____ ☐ Dreams? I felt ☐ Rested & ready for the day

I slept ☐ Well ☐ Restless ☐ Insomnia ☐ Stiff ☐ Tired ☐ Sick ☐ Sore ☐ Pain

I got up _____ times to _____ Describe _____

TODAY'S PRESCRIPTIONS AND/OR SUPPLEMENTS*

Time	Prescription/Supplement	Time	Prescription/Supplement

*WHAT YOU APPLY TO YOUR SKIN MATTERS TOO!

TODAY'S EXERCISE

Type	Time	Distance, Pounds, Repetitions, etc.
Walking		
Running		
Cycling		
Stretching		

TODAY'S ACCOMPLISHMENTS (NO MATTER HOW INSIGNIFICANT THEY MAY SEEM)

_____

_____

_____

WEIGHT	TODAY'S RECORD	DATE

Weather: ☐ Sun ☐ Clouds ☐ Rain ☐ Wind ☐ Snow Barometer:_____ Temp:_____

I have felt: ☐ Cold ☐ Hot ☐ Comfortable ☐ Mixed-bag ☐ _____

TODAY'S FOOD & DRINK

Time	Food	How I Felt After Eating

Cravings: ☐ Sweet ☐ Salty ☐ Spicy ☐ Bitter ☐ _____

Water Consumed: _____ ozs. (YOUR WEIGHT DIVIDED BY 2, EQUALS [GOAL] OUNCES TO DRINK DAILY.*)

Other Liquids Consumed & How I Felt

*HIGH ELEVATION & CHRONIC-PAIN PATIENTS, CALCULATE 1 QUART WATER PER 50 POUNDS OF WEIGHT.

BATHROOM EXPERIENCES

Bowels ☐ Constipation ☐ Diarrhea	☐ Formed ☐ Pain _____ Times	☐ Loose ☐ Pain _____ Times	☐ Cowpie ☐ Pain _____ Times	☐ Soup ☐ Pain _____ Times	☐ Odor? ☐ Painful Gas _____ Times
Urine ☐ Too Often ☐ Infrequent	☐ Clear ☐ Pain _____ Times	☐ Cloudy ☐ Pain _____ Times	☐ Light Yellow ☐ Pain _____ Times	☐ Dark Yellow ☐ Pain _____ Times	☐ Odor? ☐ Pain _____ Times

BASAL* TEMPERATURE / BLOOD-SUGAR NUMBERS / NOTES / ETC.

*The temperature that registers on an oral thermometer when it is placed under the armpit first thing in the morning before any activity.

NOTE: Your regular body temperature (TEMP) is written in the oval on the top of the left-hand side.

(TEMP)

TODAY'S SLEEP

Last night, I went to bed at _____

I fell asleep at _____ ☐ Dreams?

I slept ☐ Well ☐ Restless ☐ Insomnia

I got up _____ times to _____

Today, I woke up at _____

I felt ☐ Rested & ready for the day

☐ Stiff ☐ Tired ☐ Sick ☐ Sore ☐ Pain

Describe _____

TODAY'S PRESCRIPTIONS AND/OR SUPPLEMENTS*

Time	Prescription/Supplement	Time	Prescription/Supplement

*WHAT YOU APPLY TO YOUR SKIN MATTERS TOO!

TODAY'S EXERCISE

Type	Time	Distance, Pounds, Repetitions, etc.
Walking		
Running		
Cycling		
Stretching		

TODAY'S ACCOMPLISHMENTS (NO MATTER HOW INSIGNIFICANT THEY MAY SEEM)

_____

_____

_____

WEIGHT	TODAY'S RECORD	DATE

Weather: ☐ Sun ☐ Clouds ☐ Rain ☐ Wind ☐ Snow Barometer:_____ Temp:___H_/_L_

I have felt: ☐ Cold ☐ Hot ☐ Comfortable ☐ Mixed-bag ☐ _____

TODAY'S FOOD & DRINK

Time	Food	How I Felt After Eating

Cravings: ☐ Sweet ☐ Salty ☐ Spicy ☐ Bitter ☐ _____

Water Consumed: _____ ozs. (YOUR WEIGHT DIVIDED BY 2, EQUALS [GOAL] OUNCES TO DRINK DAILY.*)

Other Liquids Consumed & How I Felt

*HIGH ELEVATION & CHRONIC-PAIN PATIENTS, CALCULATE 1 QUART WATER PER 50 POUNDS OF WEIGHT.

BATHROOM EXPERIENCES

Bowels ☐ Constipation ☐ Diarrhea	☐ Formed ☐ Pain _____ Times	☐ Loose ☐ Pain _____ Times	☐ Cowpie ☐ Pain _____ Times	☐ Soup ☐ Pain _____ Times	☐ Odor? ☐ Painful Gas _____ Times
Urine ☐ Too Often ☐ Infrequent	☐ Clear ☐ Pain _____ Times	☐ Cloudy ☐ Pain _____ Times	☐ Light Yellow ☐ Pain _____ Times	☐ Dark Yellow ☐ Pain _____ Times	☐ Odor? ☐ Pain _____ Times

BASAL* TEMPERATURE / BLOOD-SUGAR NUMBERS / NOTES / ETC.

*The temperature that registers on an oral thermometer when it is placed under the armpit first thing in the morning before any activity.

NOTE: Your regular body temperature (TEMP) is written in the oval on the top of the left-hand side.

(TEMP)

TODAY'S SLEEP

Last night, I went to bed at _____

I fell asleep at _____ ☐ Dreams?

I slept ☐ Well ☐ Restless ☐ Insomnia

I got up _____ times to _____

Today, I woke up at _____

I felt ☐ Rested & ready for the day

☐ Stiff ☐ Tired ☐ Sick ☐ Sore ☐ Pain

Describe _____

TODAY'S PRESCRIPTIONS AND/OR SUPPLEMENTS*

Time	Prescription/Supplement	Time	Prescription/Supplement

*WHAT YOU APPLY TO YOUR SKIN MATTERS TOO!

TODAY'S EXERCISE

Type	Time	Distance, Pounds, Repetitions, etc.
Walking		
Running		
Cycling		
Stretching		

TODAY'S ACCOMPLISHMENTS (NO MATTER HOW INSIGNIFICANT THEY MAY SEEM)

_____

_____

_____

WEIGHT	TODAY'S RECORD	DATE

Weather: ☐ Sun ☐ Clouds ☐ Rain ☐ Wind ☐ Snow   Barometer:_____   Temp:_____

I have felt: ☐ Cold   ☐ Hot   ☐ Comfortable   ☐ Mixed-bag   ☐ _____

TODAY'S FOOD & DRINK

Time	Food	How I Felt After Eating

Cravings: ☐ Sweet   ☐ Salty   ☐ Spicy   ☐ Bitter   ☐ _____

Water Consumed: _____ ozs. (YOUR WEIGHT DIVIDED BY 2, EQUALS [GOAL] OUNCES TO DRINK DAILY.*)

Other Liquids Consumed & How I Felt

*HIGH ELEVATION & CHRONIC-PAIN PATIENTS, CALCULATE 1 QUART WATER PER 50 POUNDS OF WEIGHT.

BATHROOM EXPERIENCES

Bowels ☐ Constipation ☐ Diarrhea	☐ Formed ☐ Pain _____ Times	☐ Loose ☐ Pain _____ Times	☐ Cowpie ☐ Pain _____ Times	☐ Soup ☐ Pain _____ Times	☐ Odor? ☐ Painful Gas _____ Times
Urine ☐ Too Often ☐ Infrequent	☐ Clear ☐ Pain _____ Times	☐ Cloudy ☐ Pain _____ Times	☐ Light Yellow ☐ Pain _____ Times	☐ Dark Yellow ☐ Pain _____ Times	☐ Odor? ☐ Pain _____ Times

BASAL* TEMPERATURE / BLOOD-SUGAR NUMBERS / NOTES / ETC.

*The temperature that registers on an oral thermometer when it is placed under the armpit first thing in the morning before any activity.

NOTE: Your regular body temperature (TEMP) is written in the oval on the top of the left-hand side.

TEMP	TODAY'S SLEEP

Last night, I went to bed at _____   Today, I woke up at _____

I fell asleep at _____ ☐ Dreams?   I felt ☐ Rested & ready for the day

I slept ☐ Well ☐ Restless ☐ Insomnia   ☐ Stiff ☐ Tired ☐ Sick ☐ Sore ☐ Pain

I got up _____ times to _____   Describe _____

TODAY'S PRESCRIPTIONS AND/OR SUPPLEMENTS*

Time	Prescription/Supplement	Time	Prescription/Supplement

*WHAT YOU APPLY TO YOUR SKIN MATTERS TOO!

TODAY'S EXERCISE

Type	Time	Distance, Pounds, Repetitions, etc.
Walking		
Running		
Cycling		
Stretching		

TODAY'S ACCOMPLISHMENTS (NO MATTER HOW INSIGNIFICANT THEY MAY SEEM)

_____

_____

_____

| WEIGHT | TODAY'S RECORD | DATE |

Weather: ☐ Sun ☐ Clouds ☐ Rain ☐ Wind ☐ Snow   Barometer:_____   Temp:_____

I have felt: ☐ Cold   ☐ Hot   ☐ Comfortable   ☐ Mixed-bag   ☐ _____

TODAY'S FOOD & DRINK

Time	Food	How I Felt After Eating

Cravings: ☐ Sweet   ☐ Salty   ☐ Spicy   ☐ Bitter   ☐ _____

Water Consumed: OZS.   (YOUR WEIGHT DIVIDED BY 2, EQUALS [GOAL] OUNCES TO DRINK DAILY.*)

Other Liquids Consumed & How I Felt

*HIGH ELEVATION & CHRONIC-PAIN PATIENTS, CALCULATE 1 QUART WATER PER 50 POUNDS OF WEIGHT.

BATHROOM EXPERIENCES

Bowels ☐ Constipation ☐ Diarrhea	☐ Formed ☐ Pain _____ Times	☐ Loose ☐ Pain _____ Times	☐ Cowpie ☐ Pain _____ Times	☐ Soup ☐ Pain _____ Times	☐ Odor? ☐ Painful Gas _____ Times
Urine ☐ Too Often ☐ Infrequent	☐ Clear ☐ Pain _____ Times	☐ Cloudy ☐ Pain _____ Times	☐ Light Yellow ☐ Pain _____ Times	☐ Dark Yellow ☐ Pain _____ Times	☐ Odor? ☐ Pain _____ Times

BASAL* TEMPERATURE / BLOOD-SUGAR NUMBERS / NOTES / ETC.

*The temperature that registers on an oral thermometer when it is placed under the armpit first thing in the morning before any activity.

NOTE: Your regular body temperature (TEMP) is written in the oval on the top of the left-hand side.

| TEMP | TODAY'S SLEEP |

Last night, I went to bed at _____   Today, I woke up at _____

I fell asleep at _____ ☐ Dreams?   I felt ☐ Rested & ready for the day

I slept ☐ Well ☐ Restless ☐ Insomnia   ☐ Stiff ☐ Tired ☐ Sick ☐ Sore ☐ Pain

I got up _____ times to _____   Describe _____

TODAY'S PRESCRIPTIONS AND/OR SUPPLEMENTS*

Time	Prescription/Supplement	Time	Prescription/Supplement

*WHAT YOU APPLY TO YOUR SKIN MATTERS TOO!

TODAY'S EXERCISE

Type	Time	Distance, Pounds, Repetitions, etc.
Walking		
Running		
Cycling		
Stretching		

TODAY'S ACCOMPLISHMENTS (NO MATTER HOW INSIGNIFICANT THEY MAY SEEM)

_____

_____

_____

WEIGHT	TODAY'S RECORD	DATE

Weather: ☐ Sun ☐ Clouds ☐ Rain ☐ Wind ☐ Snow   Barometer:_____   Temp:_____

I have felt: ☐ Cold   ☐ Hot   ☐ Comfortable   ☐ Mixed-bag   ☐ _____

TODAY'S FOOD & DRINK

Time	Food	How I Felt After Eating

Cravings: ☐ Sweet   ☐ Salty   ☐ Spicy   ☐ Bitter   ☐ _____

Water Consumed: _____ OZS. (YOUR WEIGHT DIVIDED BY 2, EQUALS [GOAL] OUNCES TO DRINK DAILY.*)

Other Liquids Consumed & How I Felt

*HIGH ELEVATION & CHRONIC-PAIN PATIENTS, CALCULATE 1 QUART WATER PER 50 POUNDS OF WEIGHT.

BATHROOM EXPERIENCES

Bowels ☐ Constipation ☐ Diarrhea	☐ Formed ☐ Pain _____ Times	☐ Loose ☐ Pain _____ Times	☐ Cowpie ☐ Pain _____ Times	☐ Soup ☐ Pain _____ Times	☐ Odor? ☐ Painful Gas _____ Times
Urine ☐ Too Often ☐ Infrequent	☐ Clear ☐ Pain _____ Times	☐ Cloudy ☐ Pain _____ Times	☐ Light Yellow ☐ Pain _____ Times	☐ Dark Yellow ☐ Pain _____ Times	☐ Odor? ☐ Pain _____ Times

BASAL* TEMPERATURE / BLOOD-SUGAR NUMBERS / NOTES / ETC.

*The temperature that registers on an oral thermometer when it is placed under the armpit first thing in the morning before any activity.

NOTE: Your regular body temperature (TEMP) is written in the oval on the top of the left-hand side.

TEMP

TODAY'S SLEEP

Last night, I went to bed at _____

I fell asleep at _____ ☐ Dreams?

I slept ☐ Well ☐ Restless ☐ Insomnia

I got up _____ times to _____

Today, I woke up at _____

I felt   ☐ Rested & ready for the day

☐ Stiff ☐ Tired ☐ Sick ☐ Sore ☐ Pain

Describe _____

TODAY'S PRESCRIPTIONS AND/OR SUPPLEMENTS*

Time	Prescription/Supplement	Time	Prescription/Supplement

*WHAT YOU APPLY TO YOUR SKIN MATTERS TOO!

TODAY'S EXERCISE

Type	Time	Distance, Pounds, Repetitions, etc.
Walking		
Running		
Cycling		
Stretching		

TODAY'S ACCOMPLISHMENTS (NO MATTER HOW INSIGNIFICANT THEY MAY SEEM)

_____

_____

_____

WEIGHT	TODAY'S RECORD	DATE

Weather: ☐ Sun ☐ Clouds ☐ Rain ☐ Wind ☐ Snow   Barometer:_____   Temp: H___/L___

I have felt: ☐ Cold   ☐ Hot   ☐ Comfortable   ☐ Mixed-bag   ☐ _____

TODAY'S FOOD & DRINK

Time	Food	How I Felt After Eating

Cravings: ☐ Sweet   ☐ Salty   ☐ Spicy   ☐ Bitter   ☐ _____

Water Consumed: ozs.   (YOUR WEIGHT DIVIDED BY 2, EQUALS [GOAL] OUNCES TO DRINK DAILY.*)

Other Liquids Consumed & How I Felt

*HIGH ELEVATION & CHRONIC-PAIN PATIENTS, CALCULATE 1 QUART WATER PER 50 POUNDS OF WEIGHT.

BATHROOM EXPERIENCES

Bowels ☐ Constipation ☐ Diarrhea	☐ Formed ☐ Pain _____ Times	☐ Loose ☐ Pain _____ Times	☐ Cowpie ☐ Pain _____ Times	☐ Soup ☐ Pain _____ Times	☐ Odor? ☐ Painful Gas _____ Times
Urine ☐ Too Often ☐ Infrequent	☐ Clear ☐ Pain _____ Times	☐ Cloudy ☐ Pain _____ Times	☐ Light Yellow ☐ Pain _____ Times	☐ Dark Yellow ☐ Pain _____ Times	☐ Odor? ☐ Pain _____ Times

BASAL* TEMPERATURE / BLOOD-SUGAR NUMBERS / NOTES / ETC.

*The temperature that registers on an oral thermometer when it is placed under the armpit first thing in the morning before any activity.

NOTE: Your regular body temperature (TEMP) is written in the oval on the top of the left-hand side.

(TEMP)

TODAY'S SLEEP

Last night, I went to bed at _____   Today, I woke up at _____

I fell asleep at _____ ☐ Dreams?   I felt ☐ Rested & ready for the day

I slept ☐ Well ☐ Restless ☐ Insomnia   ☐ Stiff ☐ Tired ☐ Sick ☐ Sore ☐ Pain

I got up _____ times to _____   Describe _____

TODAY'S PRESCRIPTIONS AND/OR SUPPLEMENTS*

Time	Prescription/Supplement	Time	Prescription/Supplement

*WHAT YOU APPLY TO YOUR SKIN MATTERS TOO!

TODAY'S EXERCISE

Type	Time	Distance, Pounds, Repetitions, etc.
Walking		
Running		
Cycling		
Stretching		

TODAY'S ACCOMPLISHMENTS (NO MATTER HOW INSIGNIFICANT THEY MAY SEEM)

_____

_____

_____

WEIGHT	TODAY'S RECORD	DATE

Weather: ☐ Sun ☐ Clouds ☐ Rain ☐ Wind ☐ Snow   Barometer:_____   Temp:_____

I have felt: ☐ Cold ☐ Hot ☐ Comfortable ☐ Mixed-bag ☐ _____

TODAY'S FOOD & DRINK

Time	Food	How I Felt After Eating

Cravings: ☐ Sweet ☐ Salty ☐ Spicy ☐ Bitter ☐ _____

Water Consumed: _____ ozs. (YOUR WEIGHT DIVIDED BY 2, EQUALS [GOAL] OUNCES TO DRINK DAILY.*)

Other Liquids Consumed & How I Felt

*HIGH ELEVATION & CHRONIC-PAIN PATIENTS, CALCULATE 1 QUART WATER PER 50 POUNDS OF WEIGHT.

BATHROOM EXPERIENCES

Bowels ☐ Constipation ☐ Diarrhea	☐ Formed ☐ Pain ____ Times	☐ Loose ☐ Pain ____ Times	☐ Cowpie ☐ Pain ____ Times	☐ Soup ☐ Pain ____ Times	☐ Odor? ☐ Painful Gas ____ Times
Urine ☐ Too Often ☐ Infrequent	☐ Clear ☐ Pain ____ Times	☐ Cloudy ☐ Pain ____ Times	☐ Light Yellow ☐ Pain ____ Times	☐ Dark Yellow ☐ Pain ____ Times	☐ Odor? ☐ Pain ____ Times

BASAL* TEMPERATURE / BLOOD-SUGAR NUMBERS / NOTES / ETC.

*The temperature that registers on an oral thermometer when it is placed under the armpit first thing in the morning before any activity.

NOTE: Your regular body temperature (TEMP) is written in the oval on the top of the left-hand side.

(TEMP)

TODAY'S SLEEP

Last night, I went to bed at _____

I fell asleep at _____ ☐ Dreams?

I slept ☐ Well ☐ Restless ☐ Insomnia

I got up _____ times to _____

Today, I woke up at _____

I felt ☐ Rested & ready for the day

☐ Stiff ☐ Tired ☐ Sick ☐ Sore ☐ Pain

Describe _____

TODAY'S PRESCRIPTIONS AND/OR SUPPLEMENTS*

Time	Prescription/Supplement	Time	Prescription/Supplement

*WHAT YOU APPLY TO YOUR SKIN MATTERS TOO!

TODAY'S EXERCISE

Type	Time	Distance, Pounds, Repetitions, etc.
Walking		
Running		
Cycling		
Stretching		

TODAY'S ACCOMPLISHMENTS (NO MATTER HOW INSIGNIFICANT THEY MAY SEEM)

_____

_____

_____

WEIGHT	TODAY'S RECORD	DATE

Weather: ☐ Sun ☐ Clouds ☐ Rain ☐ Wind ☐ Snow   Barometer:_____   Temp:___ H ___ L

I have felt: ☐ Cold   ☐ Hot   ☐ Comfortable   ☐ Mixed-bag   ☐ _____

TODAY'S FOOD & DRINK

Time	Food	How I Felt After Eating

Cravings: ☐ Sweet   ☐ Salty   ☐ Spicy   ☐ Bitter   ☐ _____

Water Consumed: _____ OZS.   (YOUR WEIGHT DIVIDED BY 2, EQUALS [GOAL] OUNCES TO DRINK DAILY.*)

Other Liquids Consumed & How I Felt

*HIGH ELEVATION & CHRONIC-PAIN PATIENTS, CALCULATE 1 QUART WATER PER 50 POUNDS OF WEIGHT.

BATHROOM EXPERIENCES

Bowels ☐ Constipation ☐ Diarrhea	☐ Formed ☐ Pain _____ Times	☐ Loose ☐ Pain _____ Times	☐ Cowpie ☐ Pain _____ Times	☐ Soup ☐ Pain _____ Times	☐ Odor? ☐ Painful Gas _____ Times
Urine ☐ Too Often ☐ Infrequent	☐ Clear ☐ Pain _____ Times	☐ Cloudy ☐ Pain _____ Times	☐ Light Yellow ☐ Pain _____ Times	☐ Dark Yellow ☐ Pain _____ Times	☐ Odor? ☐ Pain _____ Times

BASAL* TEMPERATURE / BLOOD-SUGAR NUMBERS / NOTES / ETC.

*The temperature that registers on an oral thermometer when it is placed under the armpit first thing in the morning before any activity.

NOTE: Your regular body temperature (TEMP) is written in the oval on the top of the left-hand side.

TEMP	**TODAY'S SLEEP**
Last night, I went to bed at _____	Today, I woke up at _____
I fell asleep at _____ ☐ Dreams?	I felt ☐ Rested & ready for the day
I slept ☐ Well ☐ Restless ☐ Insomnia	☐ Stiff ☐ Tired ☐ Sick ☐ Sore ☐ Pain
I got up _____ times to _____	Describe _____

TODAY'S PRESCRIPTIONS AND/OR SUPPLEMENTS*

Time	Prescription/Supplement	Time	Prescription/Supplement

*WHAT YOU APPLY TO YOUR SKIN MATTERS TOO!

TODAY'S EXERCISE

Type	Time	Distance, Pounds, Repetitions, etc.
Walking		
Running		
Cycling		
Stretching		

TODAY'S ACCOMPLISHMENTS (NO MATTER HOW INSIGNIFICANT THEY MAY SEEM)

_____

_____

_____

WEIGHT	TODAY'S RECORD	DATE

Weather: ☐ Sun ☐ Clouds ☐ Rain ☐ Wind ☐ Snow Barometer:_____ Temp:_____

I have felt: ☐ Cold ☐ Hot ☐ Comfortable ☐ Mixed-bag ☐ _____

TODAY'S FOOD & DRINK

Time	Food	How I Felt After Eating

Cravings: ☐ Sweet ☐ Salty ☐ Spicy ☐ Bitter ☐ _____

Water Consumed: _____ ozs. (YOUR WEIGHT DIVIDED BY 2, EQUALS [GOAL] OUNCES TO DRINK DAILY.*)

Other Liquids Consumed & How I Felt

*HIGH ELEVATION & CHRONIC-PAIN PATIENTS, CALCULATE 1 QUART WATER PER 50 POUNDS OF WEIGHT.

BATHROOM EXPERIENCES

Bowels ☐ Constipation ☐ Diarrhea	☐ Formed ☐ Pain _____ Times	☐ Loose ☐ Pain _____ Times	☐ Cowpie ☐ Pain _____ Times	☐ Soup ☐ Pain _____ Times	☐ Odor? ☐ Painful Gas _____ Times
Urine ☐ Too Often ☐ Infrequent	☐ Clear ☐ Pain _____ Times	☐ Cloudy ☐ Pain _____ Times	☐ Light Yellow ☐ Pain _____ Times	☐ Dark Yellow ☐ Pain _____ Times	☐ Odor? ☐ Pain _____ Times

BASAL* TEMPERATURE / BLOOD-SUGAR NUMBERS / NOTES / ETC.

*The temperature that registers on an oral thermometer when it is placed under the armpit first thing in the morning before any activity.

NOTE: Your regular body temperature (TEMP) is written in the oval on the top of the left-hand side.

(TEMP)

TODAY'S SLEEP

Last night, I went to bed at _____

I fell asleep at _____ ☐ Dreams?

I slept ☐ Well ☐ Restless ☐ Insomnia

I got up _____ times to _____

Today, I woke up at _____

I felt ☐ Rested & ready for the day

☐ Stiff ☐ Tired ☐ Sick ☐ Sore ☐ Pain

Describe _____

TODAY'S PRESCRIPTIONS AND/OR SUPPLEMENTS*

Time	Prescription/Supplement	Time	Prescription/Supplement

*WHAT YOU APPLY TO YOUR SKIN MATTERS TOO!

TODAY'S EXERCISE

Type	Time	Distance, Pounds, Repetitions, etc.
Walking		
Running		
Cycling		
Stretching		

TODAY'S ACCOMPLISHMENTS (NO MATTER HOW INSIGNIFICANT THEY MAY SEEM)

_____

_____

_____

| WEIGHT | TODAY'S RECORD | DATE |

Weather: ☐ Sun ☐ Clouds ☐ Rain ☐ Wind ☐ Snow   Barometer:_____   Temp: H___ / L___

I have felt: ☐ Cold   ☐ Hot   ☐ Comfortable   ☐ Mixed-bag   ☐ _____

TODAY'S FOOD & DRINK

Time	Food	How I Felt After Eating

Cravings: ☐ Sweet   ☐ Salty   ☐ Spicy   ☐ Bitter   ☐ _____

Water Consumed: ozs.   (YOUR WEIGHT DIVIDED BY 2, EQUALS [GOAL] OUNCES TO DRINK DAILY.*)

Other Liquids Consumed & How I Felt

*HIGH ELEVATION & CHRONIC-PAIN PATIENTS, CALCULATE **1** QUART WATER PER **50** POUNDS OF WEIGHT.

BATHROOM EXPERIENCES

Bowels ☐ Constipation ☐ Diarrhea	☐ Formed ☐ Pain _____ Times	☐ Loose ☐ Pain _____ Times	☐ Cowpie ☐ Pain _____ Times	☐ Soup ☐ Pain _____ Times	☐ Odor? ☐ Painful Gas _____ Times
Urine ☐ Too Often ☐ Infrequent	☐ Clear ☐ Pain _____ Times	☐ Cloudy ☐ Pain _____ Times	☐ Light Yellow ☐ Pain _____ Times	☐ Dark Yellow ☐ Pain _____ Times	☐ Odor? ☐ Pain _____ Times

BASAL* TEMPERATURE / BLOOD-SUGAR NUMBERS / NOTES / ETC.

*The temperature that registers on an oral thermometer when it is placed under the armpit first thing in the morning before any activity.

NOTE: Your regular body temperature (TEMP) is written in the oval on the top of the left-hand side.

(TEMP)

TODAY'S SLEEP

Last night, I went to bed at _____

I fell asleep at _____ ☐ Dreams?

I slept ☐ Well ☐ Restless ☐ Insomnia

I got up _____ times to _____

Today, I woke up at _____

I felt ☐ Rested & ready for the day

☐ Stiff ☐ Tired ☐ Sick ☐ Sore ☐ Pain

Describe _____

TODAY'S PRESCRIPTIONS AND/OR SUPPLEMENTS*

Time	Prescription/Supplement	Time	Prescription/Supplement

*WHAT YOU APPLY TO YOUR SKIN MATTERS TOO!

TODAY'S EXERCISE

Type	Time	Distance, Pounds, Repetitions, etc.
Walking		
Running		
Cycling		
Stretching		

TODAY'S ACCOMPLISHMENTS (NO MATTER HOW INSIGNIFICANT THEY MAY SEEM)

_____

_____

_____

| WEIGHT | TODAY'S RECORD | DATE |

Weather: ☐ Sun ☐ Clouds ☐ Rain ☐ Wind ☐ Snow   Barometer:_____   Temp:_____

I have felt: ☐ Cold   ☐ Hot   ☐ Comfortable   ☐ Mixed-bag   ☐ _____

TODAY'S FOOD & DRINK

Time	Food	How I Felt After Eating

Cravings: ☐ Sweet   ☐ Salty   ☐ Spicy   ☐ Bitter   ☐ _____

Water Consumed: ozs. (YOUR WEIGHT DIVIDED BY 2, EQUALS [GOAL] OUNCES TO DRINK DAILY.*)

Other Liquids Consumed & How I Felt

*HIGH ELEVATION & CHRONIC-PAIN PATIENTS, CALCULATE 1 QUART WATER PER 50 POUNDS OF WEIGHT.

BATHROOM EXPERIENCES

Bowels ☐ Constipation ☐ Diarrhea	☐ Formed ☐ Pain _____ Times	☐ Loose ☐ Pain _____ Times	☐ Cowpie ☐ Pain _____ Times	☐ Soup ☐ Pain _____ Times	☐ Odor? ☐ Painful Gas _____ Times
Urine ☐ Too Often ☐ Infrequent	☐ Clear ☐ Pain _____ Times	☐ Cloudy ☐ Pain _____ Times	☐ Light Yellow ☐ Pain _____ Times	☐ Dark Yellow ☐ Pain _____ Times	☐ Odor? ☐ Pain _____ Times

BASAL* TEMPERATURE / BLOOD-SUGAR NUMBERS / NOTES / ETC.

*The temperature that registers on an oral thermometer when it is placed under the armpit first thing in the morning before any activity.

NOTE: Your regular body temperature (TEMP) is written in the oval on the top of the left-hand side.

(TEMP)

TODAY'S SLEEP

Last night, I went to bed at _____ Today, I woke up at _____

I fell asleep at _____ ☐ Dreams? I felt ☐ Rested & ready for the day

I slept ☐ Well ☐ Restless ☐ Insomnia ☐ Stiff ☐ Tired ☐ Sick ☐ Sore ☐ Pain

I got up _____ times to _____ Describe _____

TODAY'S PRESCRIPTIONS AND/OR SUPPLEMENTS*

Time	Prescription/Supplement	Time	Prescription/Supplement

*WHAT YOU APPLY TO YOUR SKIN MATTERS TOO!

TODAY'S EXERCISE

Type	Time	Distance, Pounds, Repetitions, etc.
Walking		
Running		
Cycling		
Stretching		

TODAY'S ACCOMPLISHMENTS (NO MATTER HOW INSIGNIFICANT THEY MAY SEEM)

_____

_____

_____

WEIGHT	TODAY'S RECORD	DATE

Weather: ☐ Sun ☐ Clouds ☐ Rain ☐ Wind ☐ Snow   Barometer:_____   Temp:____

I have felt: ☐ Cold   ☐ Hot   ☐ Comfortable   ☐ Mixed-bag   ☐ _____

TODAY'S FOOD & DRINK

Time	Food	How I Felt After Eating

Cravings: ☐ Sweet   ☐ Salty   ☐ Spicy   ☐ Bitter   ☐ _____

Water Consumed: _____ ozs.   (YOUR WEIGHT DIVIDED BY 2, EQUALS [GOAL] OUNCES TO DRINK DAILY.*)

Other Liquids Consumed & How I Felt

*HIGH ELEVATION & CHRONIC-PAIN PATIENTS, CALCULATE 1 QUART WATER PER 50 POUNDS OF WEIGHT.

BATHROOM EXPERIENCES

Bowels ☐ Constipation ☐ Diarrhea	☐ Formed ☐ Pain _____ Times	☐ Loose ☐ Pain _____ Times	☐ Cowpie ☐ Pain _____ Times	☐ Soup ☐ Pain _____ Times	☐ Odor? ☐ Painful Gas _____ Times
Urine ☐ Too Often ☐ Infrequent	☐ Clear ☐ Pain _____ Times	☐ Cloudy ☐ Pain _____ Times	☐ Light Yellow ☐ Pain _____ Times	☐ Dark Yellow ☐ Pain _____ Times	☐ Odor? ☐ Pain _____ Times

BASAL* TEMPERATURE / BLOOD-SUGAR NUMBERS / NOTES / ETC.

*The temperature that registers on an oral thermometer when it is placed under the armpit first thing in the morning before any activity.

NOTE: Your regular body temperature (TEMP) is written in the oval on the top of the left-hand side.

(TEMP)

TODAY'S SLEEP

Last night, I went to bed at _____ Today, I woke up at _____

I fell asleep at _____ ☐ Dreams? I felt ☐ Rested & ready for the day

I slept ☐ Well ☐ Restless ☐ Insomnia ☐ Stiff ☐ Tired ☐ Sick ☐ Sore ☐ Pain

I got up _____ times to _____ Describe _____

TODAY'S PRESCRIPTIONS AND/OR SUPPLEMENTS*

Time	Prescription/Supplement	Time	Prescription/Supplement

*WHAT YOU APPLY TO YOUR SKIN MATTERS TOO!

TODAY'S EXERCISE

Type	Time	Distance, Pounds, Repetitions, etc.
Walking		
Running		
Cycling		
Stretching		

TODAY'S ACCOMPLISHMENTS (NO MATTER HOW INSIGNIFICANT THEY MAY SEEM)

_____

_____

_____

| WEIGHT | TODAY'S RECORD | DATE |

Weather: ☐ Sun ☐ Clouds ☐ Rain ☐ Wind ☐ Snow   Barometer: _____   Temp: _____

I have felt: ☐ Cold ☐ Hot ☐ Comfortable ☐ Mixed-bag ☐ _____

TODAY'S FOOD & DRINK

Time	Food	How I Felt After Eating

Cravings: ☐ Sweet ☐ Salty ☐ Spicy ☐ Bitter ☐ _____

Water Consumed: _____ ozs. (YOUR WEIGHT DIVIDED BY 2, EQUALS [GOAL] OUNCES TO DRINK DAILY.*)

Other Liquids Consumed & How I Felt

*HIGH ELEVATION & CHRONIC-PAIN PATIENTS, CALCULATE 1 QUART WATER PER 50 POUNDS OF WEIGHT.

BATHROOM EXPERIENCES

Bowels ☐ Constipation ☐ Diarrhea	☐ Formed ☐ Pain _____ Times	☐ Loose ☐ Pain _____ Times	☐ Cowpie ☐ Pain _____ Times	☐ Soup ☐ Pain _____ Times	☐ Odor? ☐ Painful Gas _____ Times
Urine ☐ Too Often ☐ Infrequent	☐ Clear ☐ Pain _____ Times	☐ Cloudy ☐ Pain _____ Times	☐ Light Yellow ☐ Pain _____ Times	☐ Dark Yellow ☐ Pain _____ Times	☐ Odor? ☐ Pain _____ Times

BASAL* TEMPERATURE / BLOOD-SUGAR NUMBERS / NOTES / ETC.

*The temperature that registers on an oral thermometer when it is placed under the armpit first thing in the morning before any activity.

NOTE: Your regular body temperature (TEMP) is written in the oval on the top of the left-hand side.

SUMMARY & THOUGHTS

SUMMARY & THOUGHTS